Health Equity
and Human Rights

Important links between health and human rights are increasingly recognised, and human rights can be viewed as one of the social determinants of health. Furthermore, a human rights framework provides an excellent foundation for advocacy on health inequalities, a value-based alternative to views of health as a commodity, and the opportunity to move away from public health action being based on charity.

This text demystifies systems set up for the protection and promotion of human rights globally, regionally and nationally. It explores the use and usefulness of rights-based approaches as an important part of the toolbox available to health and welfare professionals and community members working in a variety of settings to improve health and reduce health inequities. Global in its scope, *Health Equity, Social Justice and Human Rights* presents examples from all over the world to illustrate the successful use of human rights approaches in fields such as HIV/AIDS, improving access to essential drugs, reproductive health, women's health, and improving the health of marginalised and disadvantaged groups.

Understanding human rights and their interrelationships with health and health equity is essential for public health and health promotion practitioners, as well as being important for a wide range of other health and social welfare professionals. This text is valuable reading for students, practitioners and researchers concerned with combating health inequalities and promoting social justice.

Ann Taket is Professor of Health and Social Exclusion in the School of Health and Social Development, Deakin University, Australia, and Director of the Centre for Health through Action on Social Exclusion (CHASE).

Health Equity, Social Justice and Human Rights

Ann Taket

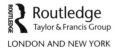

LONDON AND NEW YORK

First published 2012
by Routledge
2 Park Square, Milton Park, Abingdon, Oxon, OX14 4RN

Simultaneously published in the USA and Canada
by Routledge
711 Third Avenue, New York, NY 10017

Routledge is an imprint of the Taylor & Francis Group, an informa business

© 2012 Ann Taket for chapters 1 to 6 and 12; copyright for chapters 7 to 11 to individual authors as indicated in chapters

The right of Ann Taket to be identified as author of this work has been asserted by her in accordance with sections 77 and 78 of the Copyright, Designs and Patents Act 1988.

All rights reserved. No part of this book may be reprinted or reproduced or utilised in any form or by any electronic, mechanical, or other means, now known or hereafter invented, including photocopying and recording, or in any information storage or retrieval system, without permission in writing from the publishers.

Trademark notice: Product or corporate names may be trademarks or registered trademarks, and are used only for identification and explanation without intent to infringe.

British Library Cataloguing in Publication Data
A catalogue record for this book is available from the British Library

Library of Congress Cataloging-in-Publication Data
Taket, A. R. (Ann R.)
Health equity, social justice, and human rights / Ann Taket.
    p. ; cm. – (Routledge studies in public health)
Includes bibliographical references.
I. Title. II. Series: Routledge studies in public health.
  [DNLM: 1. Healthcare Disparities. 2. Civil Rights. 3. Health Services Accessibility. 4. Health Status Disparities. 5. Social Justice. W 84.1]
  362.1–dc23   2011045738

ISBN: 978-0-415-61374-3 (hbk)
ISBN: 978-0-415-61375-0 (pbk)
ISBN: 978-0-203-11924-2 (ebk)

Typeset in Bembo
by HWA Text and Data Management, London

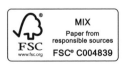

Printed and bound in Great Britain by
CPI Antony Rowe, Chippenham, Wiltshire

Contents

List of illustrations vii
List of case studies viii
List of contributors ix
Acknowledgements x
List of acronyms xi

1 Introduction 1

2 The global human rights system 7

3 Regional human rights systems 35

4 National and subnational human rights systems 56

5 Human rights and health equity 75

6 Evaluating the human rights effects of health and social policy 102

7 Addressing the sexual and reproductive health needs of adolescents in South Africa: a human rights analysis of the GOLD peer education programme 113
MELIKA CHISWELL

8 Mid-Day Meal Scheme in Madhya Pradesh: the 'Ruchikar' or Relishing Mid-Day Meal Scheme (RMDMS) 121
ARJUN SINGH

9 Tobacco Prevention Strategy in Styria, Austria: a human rights analysis 130
MICHAELA ADAMOWITSCH

10 National MindMatters Project: a retrospective human rights
    analysis   139
    CARMEL TREACY

11 The instrumental value of human rights in health   146
    BRAD CRAMMOND

12 Success or failure: how useful are rights-based approaches in
    public health?   156

    Notes on sources   170
    References   173
    Index   196

Illustrations

Figures

1.1	Multiple paths for rights-based accountability and action	5
5.1	A continuum of rights-based approaches	90
6.1	Over-inclusion: an example	107
6.2	Under-inclusion: an example	107

Tables

2.1	Summary content of the articles of the Universal Declaration of Human Rights	8
2.2	Core international human rights treaties and selected universal human rights instruments	12
2.3	Articles relating to limitation or restriction of rights	14
2.4	Four interrelated and essential elements in the right to health	18
2.5	The human rights treaty bodies	22
2.6	Selected NGOs in the global system	28
3.1	Summary features of regional human rights systems	36
3.2	Outcome of judgements and types of violation found by European Court of Human Rights, 1959–2010	50
4.1	Main features of the Paris principles for NHRIs	57
4.2	Twenty Rights in the Victorian Charter of Rights and Responsibilities	62
4.3	Members of the Bureau of the ICC and Regional Coordinating bodies	69
5.1	Possible 'ingredients' in a rights-based approach to health	80
5.2	The Integrated Nutrition and Health Project: best practices	89
6.1	The seven stage approach to human rights analysis	104
6.2	The Siracusa principles and criteria for justification of restriction of rights on grounds of protection of public health	110
9.1	Aims and objectives of TPS Styria	132
9.2	Selected aims and associated interventions and actions of TPS Styria	133

Case studies

Protecting the rights of LGBT people: NGO advocacy in action	30
The rights of the Ogoni people in the Niger Delta region	39
Mental health services in the Gambia	40
PAHO and IACHR interactions for health 1982–2007	44
Rights of people living with HIV/AIDS, IACHR Case 12.249	46
Access to palliative care in India	65
The effectiveness of the UK's Joint Committee on Human Rights	72
Domestic violence: a major public health and human rights issue	76
Health of indigenous Australians: the importance of protecting and promoting rights	78
A human rights approach to debt relief	161

Contributors

Michaela Adamowitsch is a researcher in school health promotion at the Ludwig Boltzmann Institute for health promotion research in Vienna, Austria.

Melika Chiswell is currently living in Cape Town, South Africa, and is a consultant to the nursing staff at the Desmond Tutu HIV Foundation Youth Centre Health Clinic. This clinic provides a drop-in, primary health service to young people between the ages of 12 and 22 years, the majority of whom live in the neighbouring township.

Brad Crammond is a Research Fellow at the Michael Kirby Centre for Public Health and Human Rights in the School of Public Health and Preventive Medicine at Monash University, Australia.

Arjun Singh is working as an Executive Trainee in Administration for Fortis Healthcare in India, based at Fortis Hospital, Mohali, Punjab.

Ann Taket is Professor of Health and Social Exclusion and Director of the Centre for Health through Action on Social Exclusion (CHASE) in the School of Health and Social Development, Deakin University, Australia.

Carmel Treacy is working in health promotion, specifically smoking reduction, at Neami, a non-government mental health organisation that provides support services to people with serious mental illness within a recovery framework based in Melbourne, Australia.

Acknowledgements

I would like to acknowledge with enormous thanks the interest and enthusiasm of the different cohorts of students who have taken my unit in health equity and human rights while undertaking masters degrees in public health, health promotion, social work and health and human services management at Deakin University, Australia. Their interest in the topic prompted me into the research necessary to explore the workings of the different human rights systems across the globe, at global, regional and national levels, with the aim of offering some demystification of a highly complex and interconnected web of systems. The work of four of these students is represented here in Chapters 7 to 10 and I would like to give them special thanks for joining me in this book. I would also like to thank Brad Crammond for agreeing to turn the seminar he has offered several times on my course into a chapter for inclusion.

Special thanks is due to the Unit for Health Promotion Research (Forskningsenheden for Sundhedsfremme), led by Professor Arja Aro, at the University of Southern Denmark's Esbjerg campus for offering me a wonderfully peaceful and collegial working environment during the time I spent there in September 2011. This gave the opportunity for stimulating discussions with staff and students and allowed me to complete some final editing of the manuscript.

It has proved very hard to make the final selection of what was to be included in this volume without it expanding far beyond the length agreed with the publisher. Responsibility for what was included and what was left out remains with me, and leads me to warn or promise that there is much still to explore on this topic, and that I look forward to continuing this exploration in the future.

Acronyms

ACHPR	African Commission on Human and Peoples' Rights
AFRO	WHO Regional Office for Africa
AHRC	Asian Human Rights Commission (an NGO) OR Australian Human Rights Commission (an NHRI)
AICHR	ASEAN Intergovernmental Commission on Human Rights
ALAC	Active Learning for Active Citizenship, UK programme 2004–6
ARV	Antiretroviral therapy or antiretrovirals
ASEAN	Association of Southeast Asian Nations
CAT	Convention Against Torture and other Cruel, Inhuman or Degrading Treatment or Punishment OR Committee Against Torture
CCPR	Committee on Civil and Political Rights, also known as Human Rights Committee
CED	Committee on Enforced Disappearance
CEDAW	Convention on Elimination of All Forms of Discrimination Against Women OR Committee on the Elimination of Discrimination against Women
CERD	Committee on the Elimination of Racial Discrimination
CESCR	Committee on Economic, Social and Cultural Rights
CHRAJ	Commission on Human Rights and Administrative Justice, NHRI of Ghana
CHRI	Commonwealth Human Rights Initiative, an international NGO
CIHRS	Cairo Institute for Human Rights Studies (http://www.cihrs.org)
CMW	Committee on the Protection of the Rights of All Migrant Workers and Members of their Families
CRC	Convention on the Rights of the Child OR Committee on the Rights of the Child
CRPD	Convention on the Rights of Persons with Disabilities
CSDH	Commission on the Social Determinants of Health
CVD	Cardiovascular disease
ECHR	European Convention on Human Rights
ECOSOC	Economic and Social Council, UN
EHRC	Equality and Human Rights Commission, UK's national human rights institution

EMRO	WHO Eastern Mediterranean Regional Office
EU	European Union
EURO	WHO Regional Office for Europe
FRA	European Union Agency for Fundamental Rights (http://fra.europa.eu/fraWebsite/home/home_en.htm)
GC 14	General Comment 14 on the right to health (CESCR 2000)
GLP	Global lawyers and Physicians
GoI	Government of India
HR	Human rights
HRC	Human Rights Committee, a treaty-based body within the UN system, responsible for ICCPR monitoring
HRW	Human Rights Watch, international NGO (http://www.hrw.org)
HeRWAI	Health Rights of Women Assessment Instrument
HRCl	Human Rights Council (since 2006; Commission on Human Rights before then), a charter-based body within the UN system
HREOC	Human Rights and Equal Opportunities Commission, NHRI of Australia
IACHR	Inter-American Commission on Human Rights
ICC	International Coordinating Committee of National Human Rights Institutions
ICCPR	International Covenant on Civil and Political Rights
ICERD	International Convention on the Elimination of All Forms of Racial Discrimination
ICESCR	International Covenant on Economic, Social and Cultural Rights
ICFDH	International Classification of Functioning, Disability and Health
ICHRP	International Council on Human Rights Policy, legally registered as a non-profit foundation under Swiss law since 1998. It ceased activities in December 2011, but the website (http://www.ichrp.org) is a useful archive of their work
ICPD	International Conference on Population and Development
ICRMW	International Convention on the Protection of the Rights of All Migrant Workers and Members of Their Families
IGO	Inter-Governmental Organisation OR International Governmental organisation
ILO	International Labour Office
IPR	Intellectual property rights
ISHR	International Service for Human Rights
LGTBI	Lesbian, gay, transsexual, bisexual, and intersex
MSF	Médecins Sans Frontières, international NGO
NHRC	National Human Rights Commission, India's national human rights institution
NHRI	National Human Rights Institution
NTER	Northern Territory Emergency Response
OAS	Organization of American States

OAU	Organization of African Unity
OHCHR	Office of the United Nations High Commissioner for Human Rights
OIC	Organisation of Islamic Cooperation (formerly Organisation of the Islamic Conference)
OPCAT	Optional Protocol to the Convention Against Torture
PACHR	Permanent Arab Commission on Human Rights
PAHO	Pan American Health Organization (Regional Office of WHO for the Americas)
PHM	People's Health Movement (http://www.phmovement.org)
PUCL	People's Union for Civil Liberties, India
RBA	Rights-based approach
SAPA TFAHR	Solidarity for Asian People's Advocacy Task Force on ASEAN and Human Rights
SARC	Scrutiny of Acts and Regulations Committee, Parliament of Victoria, Australia
SEARO	WHO, Regional Office for South-East Asia
SHRC	Scottish Human Rights Commission
SPT	Subcommittee on Prevention of Torture, part of the UN human rights system
STI	Sexually transmissible infection
TRIPS	Trade-Related Aspects of Intellectual Property Rights
WHA	World Health Assembly
WHO	World Health Organization
WTO	World Trade Organization
UDHR	Universal Declaration of Human Rights
UNAIDS	UNAIDS, the Joint United Nations Programme on HIV/AIDS
UNDP	United Nations Development Programme
UNEP	United Nations Environment Programme
UNESCO	United Nations Educational, Scientific and Cultural Organization
UNICEF	United Nations Children's Fund
UNHCR	United Nations High Commissioner for Refugees, the UN agency for Refugees
UPR	Universal Periodic Review
VEOHRC	Victorian Equal Opportunity and Human Rights Commission, state-level human rights body in the state of Victoria, Australia
WGNRR	Women's Global Network for Reproductive Rights

1 Introduction

Since the early 1990s there has been a growing body of work demonstrating the importance of human rights approaches within public health and other related disciplines that are concerned with seeking reductions in health inequities. There are a number of interrelated issues. First is the growing recognition of the important links between health and human rights, both direct and indirect, and across the short, medium and long term, and the considerable overlaps between human rights and the social determinants of health. Second, human rights argumentation provides an excellent foundation for advocacy on health inequities, providing a value-based alternative to views of health as a commodity to be bought and sold in the marketplace, and a move away from argumentation for public health action based on paternalistic concepts of charity. Third, human rights-based approaches are highly congruent with empowerment-based approaches now regarded as the foundation of effective health promotion, and of current thinking about the appropriate base for interactions between health professionals and their clients in many fields of practice.

Successful examples of the use of human rights approaches can be seen in fields such as HIV/AIDS, improving accessibility to essential drugs, reproductive health, women's health and improving the health of marginalised and disadvantaged groups. Knowledge of human rights is thus important at all levels in the health and social welfare arena – from the level of the interaction between an individual professional and their clients, through various levels of planning and policy-making, up to the level of global health policy and health-related policies in other sectors. Human rights analysis provides us with an important tool to help scrutinise the human rights effects (intended and unintended) of different policies, programmes and interventions, and rights-based approaches can be used to design policies and programmes that will support and promote, rather than hinder by neglect or ignorance, human rights.

Despite this growing body of significant work, there are very low levels of awareness regarding human rights, both in the public health workforce and public health students (as well as in the general public). As a small illustration, in the class of 40 commencing my course on 'Health Equity and Human Rights' in March 2010 (with students from continents across the globe, all with at least two years' public health practice), only one was aware of the Universal Declaration of Human Rights. This graphically illustrates the need for a book such as this one.

This book is distinctive in a number of aspects. First, it introduces readers to the human rights systems existing at global, regional and national levels. Secondly, it examines how rights-based approaches can be useful at all levels in the health and social welfare arenas, from the level of the interaction between an individual professional and their client up to global health policy and health-related policies in other sectors. Thirdly, it explores how human rights analysis provides an important tool to help scrutinise the human rights effects (intended and unintended) of different health-related policies, programmes and interventions, and can be used to design policies and programmes to better support reductions in health inequities. The book is global in its scope, discussing examples from all regions of the world. Finally, the book aims to encourage the reader to appreciate the value of a critical approach to health and human rights, presenting a critical appraisal of where rights-based approaches have been useful as well as an awareness of their limitations.

Health equity, social justice and human rights

> Public health should be a way of doing justice, a way of asserting the value and priority of all human life ... public health is ultimately and essentially an ethical enterprise committed to the notion that all persons are entitled to protection against the hazards of this world and to the minimisation of death and disability in society.
>
> (Beauchamp 1976: 13)

The Ottawa Charter (WHO 1986) lists social justice and equity among the prerequisites for health, alongside peace, shelter, education, food, income, a stable ecosystem and sustainable resources. The report of the Commission on the Social Determinants of Health (CSDH 2008) emphasises the importance of social justice and broad political and economic determinants in the world's health agenda (Muntaner *et al.* 2009). As Venkatapuram *et al.* (2010) discuss, the work of the Commission involved direct engagement with human rights experts and discussion of the close links between human rights and the social determinants of health; what remains contested is the extent to which the Commission's final report granted a sufficiently central role to human rights, see for example Hunt (2009), Chapman (2010) and also the discussion by Crammond in Chapter 11 of this book.

Justice, understood as fairness (see for example the *Australian Concise Oxford Dictionary*), and social justice defined as 'redistributing goods and resources to improve the situations of the disadvantaged' (Bankston 2010: 165), are most closely associated with the theory of justice expounded by liberal philosopher John Rawls (1971), and are consonant with Amartya Sen's important recent contribution on the idea of justice (Sen 2009). Sen's work is particularly valuable in terms of its focus on the issue of comparative judgements (comparing social arrangements to identify which is more or less just), rather than focusing on the question of the nature of just institutions and the behavioural norms implicated in these, as

Rawls's work did. Sen's work is also fascinating in exploring a much wider range of sources, both Western and non-Western, in support of his argumentation.

Equity means social justice or fairness: 'the term inequity has a moral and ethical dimension. It refers to differences which are unnecessary and avoidable but, in addition, are also considered unfair and unjust' (Whitehead 1990: 5). The concept of equity is inherently normative, that is, value-based, while the concept of equality, understood as 'a lack of difference', is not so. Unfortunately, the term 'health inequality' is sometimes used as a synonym for 'health inequity', perhaps because inequity is seen as having an accusatory, judgemental or morally charged tone. However, it is important to recognise that, strictly speaking, these terms are not synonymous. Social justice and fairness can also be interpreted differently by different people in different settings, so that Whitehead's definition does not provide a universal standard of measurement. Braveman and Gruskin attempt to get round this problem in offering the following definition:

> Equity in health is the absence of systematic disparities in health (or in the major social determinants of health) between groups with different levels of underlying social advantage/disadvantage – that is, wealth, power, or prestige. Inequities in health systematically put groups of people who are already socially disadvantaged (for example, by virtue of being poor, female, and/ or members of a disenfranchised racial, ethnic, or religious group) at further disadvantage with respect to their health; health is essential to wellbeing and to overcoming other effects of social disadvantage.
> (Braveman and Gruskin 2003b: 254)

This concept of health inequity, Braveman and Gruskin argue, focuses attention on the distribution of resources and other processes that drive a particular kind of health inequality – that is, a systematic inequality in health (or in its social determinants) between more and less advantaged social groups, in other words, a health inequality that is unjust or unfair. As Chapter 2 will demonstrate, equity is closely related to human rights principles. The problem is that while Braveman and Gruskin's definition appears more operationalisable, it still does not remove the element of judgement entirely; although it clarifies it by referring to social disadvantage, understood in terms of wealth, power and/or prestige. Braveman and Gruskin conclude (2003b: 257):

> Equity in health means equal opportunity to be healthy, for all population groups. Equity in health thus implies that resources are distributed and processes are designed in ways most likely to move toward equalising the health outcomes of disadvantaged social groups with the outcomes of their more advantaged counterparts. This refers to the distribution and design not only of health care resources and programmes, but of all resources, policies, and programmes that play an important part in shaping health, many of which are outside the immediate control of the health sector.

Human rights systems: global, regional, national and subnational

Since 1945, the world has seen the progressive development of a complex set of interacting human rights systems: the UN global system, various regional systems and a variety of different systems at country or lower level. Chapters 2 to 4 below explore these systems. Chapter 2 focuses on the UN global human rights system. It begins by considering the Universal Declaration of Human Rights (UDHR) and the key treaties and covenants within the UN human rights system before giving a short overview of the ongoing development of the system. Next it covers the right to health and guidance on how this is to be interpreted and examines the considerable overlap between the social determinants of health and human rights. Chapter 2 then discusses government responsibilities to respect, protect and fulfil rights and considers how the global monitoring and reporting systems assist in holding governments to account for progress in realising human rights. The chapter concludes by examining some of the key debates surrounding the global system.

Regional human rights systems are considered in Chapter 3, which begins with an overview and then considers a number of different regions and their systems in turn: Africa, the Americas, Asia-Pacific, Europe, the Middle East, and the Organisation of the Islamic Conference. Throughout the chapter an overview is given of the regional charters/statements of rights and the operation of any relevant monitoring system(s). Short case studies illustrate the operation of the different systems, particularly in relation to achievements on the right to health and the social determinants of health.

In Chapter 4, examples of different national systems are considered. The concept of the National Human Rights Institution (NHRI) is introduced first. The selection of different countries serves to illustrate some contrasts in national systems as well as some challenges in particular types of system and NHRI. Sweden, Ghana, Australia, India and Japan are considered in turn. The chapter then turns to examine NHRIs and their increasing development and integration within the global system, before concluding with an examination of the limited research that exists into the effectiveness of different aspects of national human rights systems.

As the next chapters in this book move through the different levels of human rights systems, the intersections with questions of global health governance will be considered in a number of different ways: through the operation of law and the legislature, through policy formulation and implementation, and into practice and service provision. From the 1990s onwards, the increasing pace of globalisation, accompanied by increasing economic interdependence, exemplified by the global financial crisis of 2008–9, together with increasing international movements of people and products, have increasingly demanded consideration of global health governance.

Tools for public health advocacy and action: rights-based approaches to seeking social justice and health equity

A major concern of this book is to examine the many ways that human rights approaches can be used to support health and social welfare advocacy and action

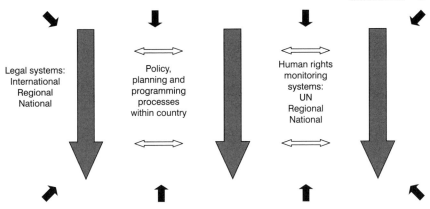

Figure 1.1 Multiple paths for rights-based accountability and action

in order to achieve social justice and health equity. Figure 1.1 depicts the different paths that may come into play, through the UN systems, through regional or national legislative routes, and through policy and programming processes. In each of these different paths, advocacy by relevant stakeholders may be highly significant in affecting the outcome.

The different pathways for accountability and action are considered in multiple places throughout the remainder of the book. In Chapter 2 the use of the UN system is considered, and the links between the social determinants of health and rights are explored; the use of legislative systems at regional level are considered in Chapter 3 and at national level in Chapter 4. In Chapter 5 the use of rights-based advocacy and human rights approaches to support policy or programme planning is examined. Here the concern is with different rights-based approaches (RBAs) that can be used in real-world processes of policy development and/or programme planning and delivery. Chapter 6 discusses methods for analysing the human rights effects of health and social policy, presenting an elaboration of a seven-stage method for human rights analysis, a desk-based activity that can be used to evaluate policies and programmes retrospectively or prospectively for their human rights implications. This seven-stage method is then applied to four contrasting policies and programmes in Chapters 7 to 10: the GOLD programme, a South African AIDS reduction initiative, is examined in Chapter 7, the mid-day meal scheme for schoolchildren in Madhya Pradesh, India, in Chapter 8, the Tobacco Prevention Strategy, Styria, Austria, in Chapter 9 and finally the National MindMatters Project, dealing with mental health promotion in secondary schools in Australia in Chapter 10. These four chapters present examples from four different continents, on diverse topics, and illustrate application of the methods of human rights analysis at both national and regional level.

Throughout Chapters 2 to 5, the uses of rights-based approaches are subject to a critical appraisal to the extent permitted by the research and evaluation evidence available. These chapters focus on where rights-based approaches have worked well, and also identify where their use has been limited or less successful. Chapters 6 to 10 illustrate the potential of human rights analysis. In Chapter 11, Crammond considers the instrumental value of human rights in health, and focuses more specifically on key important areas where rights-based approaches are of much less value, namely choosing between health programmes and between disadvantaged populations, where specific resource allocation decisions need to be made between competing priorities for treatment within and between disadvantaged populations, i.e. choosing between different interventions to treat a particular illness and choosing between interventions to be applied in different populations; often the two decisions will overlap.

WHO (2002a) posed the question 'what is the value-added of human rights in public health?' and then provided an answer in terms of eleven different elements. The first half of Chapter 12 explores the extent to which these eleven elements are evidenced in the literature. In considering the importance of human rights-based practice in public health and other health and human service sectors, this book examines the extent to which rights-based approaches provide levers for seeking actions that protect and promote public health and social welfare, and the extent to which rights-based approaches provide important tools for tackling health inequity, and supporting social justice.

This book invites the reader to consider whether the value of a rights-based approach in public health is rhetoric or reality, or more specifically, under what circumstances have rights-based approaches been useful and for what purpose? In adopting this critical questioning approach, the reader is encouraged to think about a number of different important dimensions in the context in which rights-based approaches are applied: in terms of different levels – global, regional, national, local (at various sublevels right down to including policy and practice in individual care or service provision); in terms of geography, different countries with diverse socio-economic and cultural contexts; in terms of different topics, such as HIV/AIDS, harm reduction, sexual and reproductive health, poverty; and finally, in terms of different population groups, women, children, refugees, asylum seekers, migrants, disabled people, people with mental illness. As the various chapters in the book will emphasise, achieving progress towards human rights is inextricably linked with achieving better health for all, and depends crucially on critically examining power relations within communities and societies, and how economic and political structures serve to create and recreate power relations that reinforce and reinscribe various positions of disadvantage and advantage (Taket *et al.* 2009). While it is probably self-evident that rights-based approaches are not a universal panacea for the public health professional, or any other group for that matter, it will be demonstrated that there is considerable untapped potential in their use.

2 The global human rights system

> Our contemporary human rights system is heir to demands for human dignity throughout history and across cultures. It expresses the enduring elements of the world's great philosophies, religions and cultures.
>
> (Boutros Boutros Ghali, quoted in AHRC 2009: 1)

As the quote from former UN Secretary-General Boutros Boutros Ghali emphasises, it is important to acknowledge the lengthy history of human struggles that have resulted in the creation of our contemporary human rights system. Levinson (2003) in a fascinating chronology traces the notion that all human beings have rights by virtue of being human back through history and in terms of different major religions including Buddhism, Christianity and Islam, from the earliest entry of 3000 BCE (before the common era) up until 2002; for those interested in further exploration of this history see Ishay (2008) and Moyn (2010). However, human rights were only recognised on a global scale after the Second World War. Agreement between nation-states that all people are 'born free and equal in dignity and rights' was reached in 1945 when the promotion of human rights was identified as one of the principal purposes of the newly created UN (UN 1945).

The global human rights system provides one important mechanism for holding the performance of governments to account and stimulating changes to protect, promote or fulfil human rights. This chapter focuses on the basic components of the global human rights system. It begins by looking at the Universal Declaration of Human Rights (UDHR) and then moves on to describe the key treaties and covenants in the UN human rights system, as well as the ongoing development of the system. It looks briefly at the right to health and guidance on how this is to be interpreted. The chapter then turns to examine government responsibilities to respect, protect and fulfil rights, and discusses how the global monitoring and reporting systems assist in holding governments to account for their achievements, or lack of them. The chapter concludes by reviewing briefly some of the key debates surrounding the global system.

The universal declaration of human rights (UDHR)

The UN Charter established general obligations that apply to all its member states, including respect for human rights and dignity, and in 1948 the Universal

Table 2.1 Summary content of the articles of the Universal Declaration of Human Rights

1.	All humans are free and equal	13.	Right to freedom of movement	23.	Right to work, to free choice of employment, to fair pay, to form or join a trade union
2.	No discrimination in application of rights	14.	Right to seek a safe place to live		
3.	Right to life, liberty and security	15.	Right to nationality and to change nationality	24.	Right to rest and leisure, including limitation of working hours and paid holidays
4.	No slavery				
5.	No torture or cruel or degrading treatment	16.	Right to freely chosen marriage and family		
6.	You have legal rights no matter where you are	17.	Right to own possessions	25.	Right to adequate standard of living, including food, shelter medical care and social services
		18.	Freedom of thought, conscience and religion		
7.	Everyone is equal before the law				
8.	Your human rights are protected by law	19.	Freedom of opinion and expression	26.	Right to education
		20.	Right to public assembly	27.	Right to share in culture and to copyright in works authored
9.	No arbitrary arrest, detainment or exile				
10.	Right to fair and public trial	21.	Right to participation in political affairs and public service		
				28.	A fair and free world
11.	Everyone is always innocent until proven guilty	22.	Right to social security to help you develop and to live in dignity	29.	Responsibility towards the community
				30.	No one can take away your human rights
12.	Right to privacy and not to be defamed				

Source: derived from UDHR and plain language summary prepared by the UN http://www.un.org/cyberschoolbus/humanrights/resources/plain.asp

Declaration of Human Rights (UDHR) was adopted as a common standard of achievement for all people and all nations (UN General Assembly 1948), article 1 beginning with the basic statement that: 'All human beings are born free and equal in dignity and rights'. The UDHR contains thirty articles; a brief summary of the content of each is shown in Table 2.1. An important key principle is that of non-discrimination. Article 7 is explicit: 'All are equal before the law and are entitled without any discrimination to equal protection of the law.' Other prohibitions contained in the articles of the UDHR are slavery, torture and arbitrary detention. Other articles protect freedom of expression, assembly and religion, the right to own property and the right to work and receive an education. Of particular relevance to public health is article 25, which states, in part: 'Everyone has the right to a standard of living adequate for the health and well-being of himself and his family, including food, clothing, housing and medical care and necessary social services'. A universal declaration that specified the rights of individuals was considered to be necessary to give effect to the UN Charter's provisions on human rights. The Commission on Human Rights, a standing body of the United Nations, was constituted to undertake the work of preparing the UDHR, chaired by Eleanor Roosevelt. For a fascinating analysis of the drafting process in relation particularly to article 25, see Claude and Issel (1998).

The rights contained in the UDHR are often talked about in terms of different groups or generation of rights. The so-called first generation are the civil and political rights, including the right to life, the right to liberty, the right to freedom from torture and slavery, and rights to freedom of opinion, expression and religion. Second-generation rights cover the economic and social, including rights to education, work, food, shelter, a reasonable standard of living, medical care and social services. Later on in the development of the system third- and fourth-generation rights have also been distinguished.

The UDHR is a declaration, and does not have the legal standing of a treaty. However, it was intended to provide clarification of the meaning of the terms 'fundamental freedoms' and 'human rights' appearing in the United Nations Charter, which is binding on all member states. For this it is a fundamental constitutive document of the United Nations. The declaration has served as the foundation for two binding UN human rights covenants, the International Covenant on Civil and Political Rights, and the International Covenant on Economic, Social and Cultural Rights, and the principles of the Declaration are elaborated in other international treaties considered later in this chapter.

Key features of human rights

As the UDHR makes clear, human rights are founded on respect for the dignity and worth of each person. They are universal, meaning applied equally to all people, without discrimination. They are also inalienable, meaning that no one can have his or her human rights taken away; they can be limited in specific situations (for example, the right to liberty can be limited if a person is found guilty of a crime by a court of law), and this is considered further in the next section.

Perhaps the most important feature of human rights is the notion of universality: meaning that human rights are the rights of *all* human beings. In other words, the most important right of all is everyone's right to human rights. The universality of human rights implies that human rights are fundamental to every type of society. In this way, everyone has the same basic human rights. Individuals may exercise different rights, or exercise the same rights differently, depending on which group they belong to within society. Relevant different groups include women and children, as well as groups defined by culture, ethnicity or religion. Even if the form or content of human rights changes over time, the principle of their universality remains constant.

Human rights as a set are indivisible, interrelated and interdependent, individual human rights do not exist in isolation of each other. As a consequence, it is insufficient to respect some human rights and not others; if one right is violated, this will often also affect respect for several other rights. This does not however mean that rights always reinforce one another positively. Sometimes they complement one another and at other times there is tension or conflict between them. Sometimes this is a direct contradiction, for example the right to cultural or religious practice for one group may clash with the right not to be discriminated against on certain grounds for other groups. Tensions between rights may also occur when they are effectively in competition with each other for limited resources, for example the rights to a healthy environment, to an education, to health care or to welfare benefits. A fourth feature of human rights is that they are inabrogable, meaning that they cannot voluntarily be given up or traded for other privileges.

Two different types of rights are distinguished: absolute and relative. Absolute rights are those where no restrictions or limitations may be placed on them, even if argued as necessary for some public good; absolute rights include: the right to be free from torture, slavery or servitude; the right to a fair trial; the right to freedom of thought. The right to life is *not* absolute, what is forbidden is arbitrary deprivation of life. Note also that the right to freedom of thought/opinion and the right to hold any opinion do not include unlimited right to free expression of opinion. It is qualified by certain restrictions or limitations, those which are provided by law and are necessary: (a) for respect of the rights or reputations of others; (b) for the protection of national security or of public order (*ordre public*), or of public health or morals. This illustrates the complex interdependence that exists between the achievement of rights of different groups within the same community, and some of the articles in the conventions provide guidance on when rights can justifiably be restricted. This is discussed further when these other human rights instruments are considered. The question of when rights can justifiably be restricted or limited is taken up in a later section in this chapter.

The ongoing development of the system

Once the UDHR had been put into place, work began to develop more explicit human rights standards and to set in place specific monitoring and reporting mechanisms. This ushered in an extended period of development that resulted in the two International Covenants, of Civil and Political Rights, and of Economic, Cultural and Social Rights, that were adopted in 1966; the UDHR together with the ICCPR and ICESCR are referred to as the 'International Bill of Human Rights'. Building on these, other instruments have been developed, expanding on rights for particular population groups and issues. The key features of the process can be illuminated by considering the creation of the Convention on the Rights of Persons with Disabilities (CRPD), one of the latest conventions to be adopted. This began with the passing of resolution 56/168 on 19 December 2001, by the United Nations General Assembly which established an Ad Hoc Committee to negotiate for a comprehensive and integral international convention to promote and protect the rights and dignity of persons with disabilities. The first meeting of this committee was held from 29 July to 9 August 2002. Drafting of the text began in May 2004, and the final text was agreed in the eighth and final session of the Ad Hoc Committee held from 14 to 25 August 2006. Delegates to the Committee represented NGOs, governments, national human rights institutes and international organisations. This was the first time that NGOs had actively participated in the formulation of a human rights instrument.

This continuing development of human rights emphasises their discursive and evolving nature. Although the UDHR can be seen as an impressive and inspirational achievement, with significant social justice implications, it is important to recognise that the language used would be rather different if the text were being authored today, in that a more gender-neutral formulation would be highly likely.

A convention (sometimes called a covenant) is a binding treaty, coming into force upon ratification by a certain number of states. Once an instrument is adopted by the General Assembly of the UN or other relevant committee/grouping, it is then opened for signature; countries sign the treaty to indicate their willingness to proceed through necessary steps to be bound by the treaty. Where the signature is subject to ratification, acceptance or approval, the signature does not establish the consent to be bound, it signals *intention*, not *commitment*. However, it is a means of authentication and expresses the willingness of the signatory state to continue the treaty-making process. The signature qualifies the signatory state to proceed to ratification, acceptance or approval. It also creates an obligation to refrain, in good faith, from acts that would defeat the object and the purpose of the treaty. So, ratification or accession are the terms used when a country indicates its agreement to be bound by a treaty. If one were cynical, one might suspect that this allows some countries to maintain a façade of compliance by remaining as signatories for a long period of time or even indefinitely, for example the ICESCR has been signed but not ratified (as at 21 January 2011) by Belize, Comoros, Cuba, Sao Tome and Principe, South Africa and the USA. The comment made by Cuba in relation to its signature offers us a specific explanation in referring to the difficulties of making progress while being the subject of an economic blockade. Once an instrument has come into force, the term 'accession' is used for further countries who agree to be bound by the instrument: this is equivalent to ratification. Table 2.2 shows the major human rights instruments and, for each, the date of adoption, and the date the instrument came into force.

Key treaties and covenants in the UN human rights systems

More than twenty multilateral human rights treaties have been formulated since 1948. As discussed above these create legally binding obligations on those countries that have ratified them. Particularly important treaties are the International Covenant on Civil and Political Rights, ICCPR, and the International Covenant on Economic, Social and Cultural Rights, ICESCR; both of these were adopted by the UN General Assembly on 16 December 1966. The creation of two covenants, with much overlap (and even more interrelationship) but distinct focuses, deserves some comment. Part of the reason for their division flows from the history of the cold war, but there is also the distinct form and nature of the two sets of rights they contain (Gruskin *et al.* 2005). Civil and political rights can be seen as 'negative' rights or freedoms, generally requiring states *not* to interfere in the affairs of their citizens (e.g. privacy, freedom of expression, thought and religion, freedom of movement and assembly, and freedom from torture, arbitrary arrest and discrimination); these are the rights are often referred to as 'first-generation' rights. In contrast, economic, social and cultural rights can be considered 'positive' rights, requiring states actively to implement measures to secure them (e.g. right to a clean environment, rights to education, health, welfare assistance); these are the so-called second-generation

Table 2.2 Core international human rights treaties and selected universal human rights instruments

Acronym	Full name	Date of adoption	Date of coming into force
Core international human rights treaties			
ICERD	International Convention on the Elimination of All Forms of Racial Discrimination	21 Dec 1965	4 Jan 1969
ICCPR	International Covenant on Civil and Political Rights ★	16 Dec 1966	23 Mar 1976
ICESCR	International Covenant on Economic, Social and Cultural Rights ★	16 Dec 1966	3 Jan 1976
CEDAW	Convention on the Elimination of All Forms of Discrimination against Women ★	18 Dec 1979	3 Sept 1981
CAT	Convention against Torture and Other Cruel, Inhuman or Degrading Treatment or Punishment ★	10 Dec 1984	26 June 1987
CRC	Convention on the Rights of the Child ★	20 Nov 1989	2 Sept 1990
ICRMW	International Convention on the Protection of the Rights of All Migrant Workers and Members of Their Families	18 Dec 1990	1 July 2003
CRPD	Convention on the Rights of Persons with Disabilities ★	13 Dec 2006	3 May 2008
CPPED	International Convention for the Protection of All Persons from Enforced Disappearance	20 Dec 2006	23 Dec 2010
Selected universal human rights instruments †			
	Convention relating to the Status of Refugees	28 July 1951	22 Apr 1954
	Convention relating to the Status of Stateless Persons	28 Sept 1954	6 June 1960
	Protocol relating to the Status of Refugees	16 Dec 1966	4 Oct 1967
	Convention on the Reduction of Statelessness	30 Aug 1961	13 Dec 1975
	Declaration on the Human Rights of Individuals Who are not Nationals of the Country in which They Live	13 Dec 1985	
	Indigenous and Tribal Peoples Convention	27 June 1989	5 Sept 1991
	United Nations Principles for Older Persons	16 Dec 1991	
	Declaration on the Rights of Persons Belonging to National or Ethnic, Religious and Linguistic Minorities	18 Dec 1992	
	Declaration on the Rights of Indigenous Peoples	2 Oct 2007	

★ Indicates that the covenant or convention concerned has one or more optional protocols that were adopted and came into force at later dates.
† Only a very limited selection has been given here, a full list can be found on http://www.ohchr.org/ , by selecting human rights instruments

Source: compiled from information given on http://www.ohchr.org/ and http://treaties.un.org/

rights. The Convention of the Rights of the Child, the first human rights treaty to be opened for signature after the end of the cold war includes civil, political, economic and social rights considerations not only within the same treaty, but within the same right – for example in article 6 of the CRC.

More recently, during the closing decades of the twentieth century, a third generation of collective rights has been identified, to some extent this arises out of Asian critiques of the first- and second-generation rights as not responding adequately to cultures with more collective than individual norms. These rights include the right to economic development, the right to benefit from world trade and economic growth and environmental rights. This set of rights is less well represented in treaties and conventions, and remains an important area for future development. The issue is returned to in the last section of this chapter. Sometimes a fourth generation of rights is distinguished to cover the collective rights of indigenous peoples (e.g. Messer 1993; Brinton Lykes 2001; Broderstad 2010), at other times the term 'fourth generation' is used to refer to information or communication rights (Neshat 2004; Shade 2004), and at still other times to refer to intergenerational justice or the rights of future generations (Grech 2009).

When can rights be restricted or limited?

The interdependence of rights has been noted earlier. This subsection looks at the question of what constitutes 'valid' or justifiable limitations on human rights. The UDHR and the two covenants both discuss the issue, setting out the circumstances in which limitation of rights can be justified. They do this in two different ways, first in general articles, and then specifically in relation to particular rights. Relevant articles from the UDHR, ICCPR and ICESCR are shown in Table 2.3. The form of the limitation varies as shown in the table; of particular interest are those rights that may be limited on public health grounds, including freedom of movement and association, but also freedom of expression and freedom to manifest one's religion or beliefs.

ICCPR article 4 contains a very important exclusion, that of any limitation that involves discrimination on specific grounds. The corresponding article in the ICESCR is perhaps less precise (and thus less useful) in its formulation. Recognising the difficulty of the judgements that need to be exercised in deciding whether a specific limitation of rights is justified or not, work was carried out to formulate a series of principles to help decide whether limitations are just or not. This resulted in the five Siracusa principles (ECOSOC 1984). These state that, when a government limits the exercise or enjoyment of a right, this action must be taken as a last resort and will only be considered legitimate if the following five criteria are met: the restriction is provided for and carried out in accordance with the law; the restriction is in the interest of a legitimate objective of general interest; the restriction is strictly necessary in a democratic society to achieve this objective; there are no less intrusive and restrictive means available to reach the same goal; and the restriction is not imposed arbitrarily, i.e. in an unreasonable or otherwise discriminatory manner. In the case of restriction on the grounds of protection of public health, Gostin (quoted in Coker 2001) suggests the following specific criteria for use: risk posed should

Table 2.3 Articles relating to limitation or restriction of rights

Treaty and article	Text
UDHR, Article 29	1 Everyone has duties to the community in which alone the free and full development of his personality is possible. 2 In the exercise of his rights and freedoms, everyone shall be subject only to such limitations as are determined by law solely for the purpose of securing due recognition and respect for the rights and freedoms of others and of meeting the just requirements of morality, public order and the general welfare in a democratic society. 3 These rights and freedoms may in no case be exercised contrary to the purposes and principles of the United Nations.
ICCPR, Article 4	i [I]n time of public emergency which threatens the life of the nation and the existence of which is officially proclaimed, the States Parties to the present Covenant may take measures derogating from their obligations under the present Covenant to the extent strictly required by the exigencies of the situation, provided that such measures are not inconsistent with their other obligations under international law and do not involve discrimination solely on the grounds of race, colour, sex, language, religion or social origin.
ICESCR, Article 4	The States Parties to the present Covenant recognize that, in the enjoyment of those rights provided by the State in conformity with the present Covenant, the State may subject such rights only to such limitations as are determined by law only in so far as this may be compatible with the nature of these rights and solely for the purpose of promoting the general welfare in a democratic society.
ICCPR, Article 12 Freedom of movement	… not be subject to any restrictions except those which are provided by law, are necessary to protect national security, public order (ordre public), public health or morals or the rights and freedoms of others
ICCPR, Article 18, para 3 Freedom to manifest one's religion or beliefs	Freedom to manifest one's religion or beliefs may be subject only to such limitations as are prescribed by law and are necessary to protect public safety, order, health, or morals or the fundamental rights and freedoms of others.
ICCPR, Article 19, para 2 freedom of expression	The exercise of the rights provided for in paragraph 2 of this article carries with it special duties and responsibilities. It may therefore be subject to certain restrictions, but these shall only be such as are provided by law and are necessary: (a) For respect of the rights or reputations of others; (b) For the protection of national security or of public order (ordre public), or of public health or morals.
ICCPR, Article 21 Peaceful assembly Article 22 Freedom of association with others, including the right to form and join trade unions	No restrictions may be placed on the exercise of this right other than those imposed in conformity with the law and which are necessary in a democratic society in the interests of national security or public safety, public order (ordre public), the protection of public health or morals or the protection of the rights and freedoms of others.
ICESCR, Article 8 Trade unions	… subject to no limitations other than those prescribed by law and which are necessary in a democratic society in the interests of national security or public order or for the protection of the rights and freedoms of others;

Source: http://www.ohchr.org/

be demonstrable and significant; proposed interventions should be demonstrably effective; approach should be cost-effective; sanctions should be least restrictive necessary; policy should be fair and non-discriminatory.

Within public health, infectious diseases present one of the clearest examples where restrictions of human rights need to be considered. The HIV/AIDS pandemic, as well as SARS (Lam *et al.* 2003) and swine flu (Pada and Tambyah 2011), have provided many instances where restrictions have been introduced affecting rights to freedom of movement. Some websites (e.g. www.hivtravel.org) give information about restrictions on the freedom of movement for people who are HIV positive, including requirements for HIV testing prior to entry for different countries. Application of the public health version of the Siracusa principles suggests that none of these restrictions can be justified on public health grounds.

Cuba as a country has come in for considerable international criticism in relation to its response to HIV/AIDS, in particular for its practice, in the early stages of the pandemic, of quarantining those who were HIV positive. This criticism persists to the present day, for example, according to the About Aids website (http://aids.about.com) on 11 August 2010: 'Foreign students, foreign workers and long-term foreign residents are screened for HIV; people found to be HIV positive are reportedly repatriated'. Anderson (2009) presents a very careful rights-based analysis of Cuba's approach to HIV/AIDS; he concludes that, while Cuba's quarantine period was unnecessarily prolonged in the 1980s, this policy did not display discrimination in only targeting particular groups (men who have sex with men) given the state of knowledge at the time. He identifies that selective criticism of the Cuban programme has painted an inaccurate picture overall.

In applying the public health version of the Siracusa principles given above, Gostin and Lazzarini (1997: 66), talking about HIV, stress the importance of careful determination of significant risk:

> Significant risk must be determined on a case by case basis through fact specific individual inquiries. Blanket rules or generalizations about a class of persons with HIV infection do not suffice. The risk must be 'significant', not merely speculative or remote. For example, theoretically, a person could transmit HIV by biting, spitting, or splattering blood, but the actual risk is extremely low (approaching zero). Likewise, an HIV-positive health professional who does not perform deeply invasive procedures is highly unlikely to transmit HIV to a patient. Present knowledge does not support screening or excluding that person from the health care profession because, lacking a real and substantial possibility of HIV transmission, such policies do not meet the significant risk test.
>
> (Gostin and Lazzarini 1997: 66)

More recently, Bisaillon (2010) analyses the human rights consequences of the mandatory HIV screening policy for newcomers to Canada, finding a number of problems including unclear objectives and goals for the programme, and instances of stigmatisation and discrimination within its operation. Her paper identifies recommendations for addressing the human rights consequences of the policy.

The 'right to health'

> The enjoyment of the highest attainable standard of health is one of the fundamental rights of every human being ...
> (Preamble to the WHO Constitution)

One particularly important right for public health practitioners is the so-called right to health. Not only is it directly stated in the preamble to the WHO constitution, article 25 of the UDHR mentions 'health and wellbeing', and article 12 of the ICESCR is then more explicit:

1 The States Parties to the present Covenant recognise the right of everyone to the enjoyment of the highest attainable standard of physical and mental health.
2 The steps to be taken by the States Parties to the present Covenant to achieve the full realisation of this right shall include those necessary for:
   a) the provision for the reduction of the stillbirth rate and of infant mortality and for the healthy development of the child;
   b) the improvement of all aspects of environmental and industrial hygiene;
   c) the prevention, treatment and control of epidemic, endemic, occupational and other diseases;
   d) the creation of conditions which would assure to all, medical service and medical attention in the event of sickness.

This explicit recognition of the highest attainable standard of health as a 'human right' as opposed to a good or commodity with a charitable construct provides a very powerful basis for public health and health promotion advocacy. It is important to note that the Covenant mentions explicitly both mental health and physical health, but does not include social health (as the WHO Constitution did); many have seen this as unfortunate. Other international human rights instruments also address the right to health, both generally and in relation to specific groups, for example: ICERD article 5(e)(iv); CEDAW articles 11(1)(f), 12 and 14(2)(b); CRC article 24; ICRMW articles 28, 43(e) and 45(c); CRPD article 25. In thinking about the implications of the right to health, Mary Robinson, a previous United Nations High Commissioner for Human Rights, expresses some very important key features:

> The right to health does not mean the right to be healthy, nor does it mean that poor governments must put in place expensive health services for which they have no resources. But it does require governments and public authorities to put in place policies and action plans which will lead to available and accessible health care for all in the shortest possible time. To ensure that this happens is the challenge facing both the human rights community and public health professionals.
> (WHO 2002a: 9)

In helping countries move towards the right to health, the monitoring committee responsible for the ICESCR formulated General Comment 14 (CESCR 2000), and the UN Office of the High Commissioner for Human Rights and WHO have produced a fact sheet on the right to health (WHO 2008a). One of the key normative points about the right to health is that it is held to extend to the underlying determinants of health (CESCR 2000: paragraphs 4, 10 and 11); this thus specifically includes many of the other rights that have considerable overlaps with the social and cultural determinants of health, see below. Also important is the participation of population in all health-related decision-making at community, national and international levels (CESCR 2000: paragraphs 11, 17, 34 and 54).

As General Comment 14 makes clear, the right to health is *not* to be understood as the 'right to be healthy', this being impossible to achieve or guarantee. The notion of 'the highest attainable standard of health' in ICESCR article 12.1 takes into account both the individual's biological and socio-economic preconditions and a state's available resources. There are a number of aspects which cannot be addressed solely within the relationship between states and individuals; in particular, good health cannot be ensured by a state, nor can states provide protection against every possible cause of human ill health. Genetic factors, individual susceptibility to ill health and the adoption of unhealthy or risky lifestyles all influence an individual's health. The right to health contains both freedoms and entitlements. The freedoms include: the right to control one's health and body, including sexual and reproductive freedom, and the right to be free from interference, such as the right to be free from torture, non-consensual medical treatment and experimentation. Entitlements include the right to a system of health protection which provides equality of opportunity for people to enjoy the highest attainable level of health and the participation of the population in all health-related decision-making at the community, national and international levels.

The right to health includes the right of access to a variety of facilities, goods, services and conditions necessary for the realisation of the highest attainable standard of health. The Committee interprets the right to health as an inclusive right extending not only to timely and appropriate health care, but also to the underlying determinants of health, such as access to safe and potable water and adequate sanitation, an adequate supply of safe food, nutrition and housing, healthy occupational and environmental conditions, and access to health-related education and information, including on sexual and reproductive health.

According to General Comment 14, the right to health contains four interrelated and essential elements: availability, accessibility, acceptability and quality. These are expanded on in Table 2.4. Within some of the elements, there is the potential for tensions or outright conflicts. For example, note the potential conflicts that may occur in item (c) on acceptability through differences between medical ethics and the notions of cultural appropriateness held by particular groups. The notion of core obligations is also important. These were introduced in General Comment 3 on 'The nature of States parties' obligations' (CESCR 1990) which confirms that states parties have a *core obligation* to ensure the satisfaction of, at the very least, minimum essential levels of each of the rights in the Covenant. General Comment 14 then expands by stating that the core obligations of the right to health include those given as the essential components of primary health care enshrined in the Alma Ata

Table 2.4 Four interrelated and essential elements in the right to health

(a) Availability	Functioning facilities, goods and services, as well as programmes, have to be available in sufficient quantity. The precise nature of the facilities, goods and services will vary depending on numerous factors, including the developmental level of the country concerned. They will include, however, the underlying determinants of health, such as safe and potable drinking water and adequate sanitation facilities, hospitals, clinics and other health-related buildings, trained medical and professional personnel receiving domestically competitive salaries, and essential drugs, as defined by the WHO Action Programme on Essential Drugs.
(b) Accessibility	Health facilities, goods and services have to be accessible to everyone without discrimination, within the jurisdiction of the country. Accessibility has four overlapping dimensions: (i) Non-discrimination: accessible to all, especially the most vulnerable or marginalized sections of the population, in law and in fact, without discrimination on any of the prohibited grounds. (ii) Physical accessibility: within safe physical reach for all sections of the population, especially vulnerable or marginalized groups, such as ethnic minorities and indigenous populations, women, children, adolescents, older persons, persons with disabilities and persons with HIV/AIDS. Accessibility also implies that medical services and underlying determinants of health, such as safe and potable water and adequate sanitation facilities, are within safe physical reach, including in rural areas. This also includes adequate access to buildings for persons with disabilities. (iii) Economic accessibility (affordability): must be affordable for all. Payment for health-care services, as well as services related to the underlying determinants of health, has to be based on the principle of equity, ensuring that these services, whether privately or publicly provided, are affordable for all, including socially disadvantaged groups. Equity demands that poorer households should not be disproportionately burdened with health expenses as compared to richer households. (iv) Information accessibility: accessibility includes the right to seek, receive and impart information and ideas concerning health issues. However, accessibility of information should not impair the right to have personal health data treated with confidentiality.
(c) Acceptability	Services must be respectful of medical ethics and culturally appropriate, i.e. respectful of the culture of individuals, minorities, peoples and communities, sensitive to gender and life-cycle requirements, as well as being designed to respect confidentiality and improve the health status of those concerned.
(d) Quality	As well as being culturally acceptable, health facilities, goods and services must also be scientifically and medically appropriate and of good quality. This requires, inter alia, skilled medical personnel, scientifically approved and unexpired drugs and hospital equipment, safe and potable water, and adequate sanitation.

Source: Derived from paragraph 12 (CESCR 2000)

declaration (CESCR 2000: paragraphs 43 and 44). In the case of HIV/AIDS, more specific elaborations have been given elsewhere by WHO and UN Human Rights Commission (World Health Assembly 2000; Commission on Human Rights 2001) to ensure provision and affordability of drugs.

The appearance of the content of the Alma Ata declaration within General Comment 14 was a direct result of WHO's re-engagement with the developing global human rights system from 1973 onwards (Meier 2010). Meier provides a fascinating analysis of WHO's involvement with the evolving global human rights system over the period 1948 to 1980. He distinguishes three separate periods. During the first of these, 1948–52, WHO was closely involved with the initial stages of discussion and drafting for what was to become the ICESCR, arguing for the broad understanding of health given in WHO's constitution, and for explicit consideration of health promotion. During the second period, under different leadership at WHO, as the drafting process was completed, WHO remained on the sidelines, concentrating on a biomedical approach with vertical disease-specific approaches to international public health, and the resulting article 12 in the ICESCR reflects a much narrower conception of health. By the 1973 election of Halfdan Mahler as Director-General of WHO, the epidemiological transition and the recognition of the challenges of non-communicable diseases, coupled with the failure of vertical disease-based programmes in cases such as malaria, had created a different climate and WHO re-engaged with human rights, initially through espousing a needs-based approach to health development through primary health care, and resulting, in 1978, in article 1 of the Alma Ata declaration:

> The Conference strongly reaffirms that health, which is a state of complete physical, mental and social wellbeing, and not merely the absence of disease or infirmity, is a fundamental human right and that the attainment of the highest possible level of health is a most important world-wide social goal whose realization requires the action of many other social and economic sectors in addition to the health sector.

The Alma Ata declaration is seen by Meier (2010) to represent a rights-based approach to health.

Throughout the foregoing and specifically in discussion of accessibility (section b in Table 2.4), the right to freedom from discrimination has been argued as particularly important, as Jonathan Mann, Director of the Global Programme on HIV/AIDS from 1986 to 1990 and founding Director of the François-Xavier Bagnoud Center for Health and Human Rights at Harvard University, put it:

> Public health practice is heavily burdened by the problem of inadvertent discrimination. For example, outreach activities may 'assume' that all populations are reached equally by a single, dominant-language message on television; or analysis 'forgets' to include health problems uniquely relevant to certain groups, like breast cancer or sickle cell disease; or a problem 'ignores' the actual response capability of different population groups, as when lead poisoning warnings are

given without concern for financial ability to ensure lead abatement. Indeed, inadvertent discrimination is so prevalent that all public health policies and programmes should be considered discriminatory until proven otherwise, placing the burden on public health to affirm and ensure its respect for human rights.

(Mann 1997: 9)

Looking at international recognition of the right to health, Kinney (2001) summarises the position in 2000 in terms of three different measures: 142 out of 193 countries have ratified the ICESCR, 109 have a recognition in their national constitutions and 83 have ratified a regional treaty with a right to health. More recently, SEARO (2011) examined the right to health in the constitutions of the eleven countries in the South-East Asia Region of WHO, finding it enshrined in the constitutions of six countries, while in the other five the provision is more limited – in terms of the right to certain types of health care. Backman *et al.* (2008) examine achievement in relation to the right to health in terms of a variety of different indicators for 194 countries; they find a very mixed picture of achievement; for example, only 56 of the 160 countries that have ratified ICESCR have legally recognised the right to health.

Human rights and the social and cultural determinants of health

… there is a powerful synergy between health and rights. By design, neglect or ignorance, health policies and programs can promote and protect or conversely restrict and violate human rights. Similarly, the promotion, protection, restriction or violation of human rights can have direct impacts on health.

(Brundtland, 2005: 61)

In this quote Gro Harlem Brundtland (the Director-General of WHO in 2005) makes reference to the understanding that the major determinants of better health lie outside the health system, and include the fulfilment of an array of rights that are relevant to the right to health in the understanding of General Comment 14. Health policies, programmes and practices, in and of themselves, can promote and protect OR restrict and violate human rights, by design, neglect or ignorance, and Chapter 6 discusses the human rights analysis that can be carried out in order to explore the rights implications of policies and programmes. In terms of the influence of human rights on health, first, human rights violations can directly affect health: for example, harmful traditional practices, torture, slavery, violence against women and children; such effects on health can be in the short, medium and/or long term. Secondly, vulnerability to ill health can be reduced through the promotion of human rights, for example of the right to health, to education, to food and nutrition and to freedom from discrimination. Promotion, protection and restriction or violations of human rights all have both direct and indirect impacts on health and wellbeing; these can also be proximal or distal. Since the 1980s, the HIV/AIDS pandemic and reproductive and sexual health concerns in particular have been instrumental in clarifying the interrelationships between health and human rights (Gruskin et al. 2007). This is considered further in Chapter 5.

It can be seen that the links between human rights and the social and cultural determinants of health are many and direct (a detailed mapping is given in Taket 2012). Rights to education, employment and occupation, food, shelter, water, sanitation, safety, freedom of movement and expression (see Table 2.1) include many of the factors understood as social determinants of health (CSDH 2008). Thus action taken to support a broad range of human rights can be understood as supporting health, and similarly action on many social determinants of health, with attention to moving towards health equity, is also action to support human rights.

Global monitoring and reporting systems

Governments are responsible not only for not directly violating rights but also for ensuring the conditions which enable individuals to realise their rights as fully as possible. This is understood as an obligation to respect, protect and fulfil rights. By ratifying the different human rights instruments, governments also acquire reporting requirements which enable the monitoring of progress within the UN human rights system. There are nine core human rights treaties, corresponding to these are nine bodies/committees that monitor the performance of those countries who have ratified or acceded to the treaty in their efforts to comply with the treaty's provisions, see Table 2.5. Full details can be found on the OHCHR website, www.ohchr.org. The dates of the first meetings of the different treaty bodies shown in Table 2.5 illustrate the development of the system over time; the treaty bodies are listed in order of the year of their first meeting.

A central feature of the monitoring process is that all committees have reporting requirements. Each country is required first to lodge a report with the committee (usually referred to as 'country reports') detailing the status of its compliance with the treaty in question *at the time of the country becoming a party to the treaty*. Subsequently, countries are required to lodge supplementary reports at four- or five-yearly intervals. In addition, the committees conduct hearings with government representatives during which aspects of country reports are examined in detail. NGOs may submit 'Alternative' Reports to the relevant committees; these may also be referred to during the committee hearings. Each treaty body receives secretariat support from the Human Rights Treaties Branch of OHCHR in Geneva.

All committees have the capacity to issue 'General Comments'. The object of these General Comments is to provide countries with guidance in their efforts to meet their treaty obligations. This guidance is gleaned from the committees' experiences in reviewing the country reports submitted to them. The General Comments are intended to assist countries in this regard by providing greater detail about what the requirements are and how best they can be met. Where appropriate, the General Comments also draw upon the committees' own published opinions in respect of individual communications or cases. They cover such matters as expanded definitions of key terms, the use of reservations and derogations, and reporting requirements and standards.

Table 2.5 The human rights treaty bodies

Treaty body and role	Year of first meeting
The Committee on the Elimination of Racial Discrimination (CERD) monitors implementation of the International Convention on the Elimination of All Forms of Racial Discrimination (1965)	1970
The Human Rights Committee (CCPR) monitors implementation of the International Covenant on Civil and Political Rights (1966) and its optional protocols	1976
The Committee on the Elimination of Discrimination Against Women (CEDAW) monitors implementation of the Convention on the Elimination of All Forms of Discrimination against Women (1979) and its optional protocol (1999)	1982
The Committee on Economic, Social and Cultural Rights (CESCR) monitors implementation of the International Covenant on Economic, Social and Cultural Rights (1966)	1985
The Committee Against Torture (CAT) monitors implementation of the Convention against Torture and Other Cruel, Inhuman or Degrading Treatment (1984)	1988
The Committee on the Rights of the Child (CRC) monitors implementation of the Convention on the Rights of the Child (1989) and its optional protocols (2000)	1991
The Committee on Migrant Workers (CMW) monitors implementation of the International Convention on the Protection of the Rights of All Migrant Workers and Members of Their Families (1990)	2004
The Committee on the Right of Persons with Disabilities (CRPD) monitors implementation of the International Convention on the Rights of Persons with Disabilities (2006)	2009
The Committee on Enforced Disappearance (CED) monitors implementation of the International Convention for the Protection of All Persons from Enforced Disappearance (2006)	2011

There are two levels at which the committees may receive complaints (usually called 'communications') that human rights violations have occurred. First, they may receive communications from governments, that is, where one government alleges that another has violated rights protected by a treaty to which it is a party. It is not surprising that this mechanism is rarely used, given diplomatic reluctance between governments to accuse each other of breaches in their human rights obligations. Secondly, a committee may be empowered to receive and consider individual communications, that is, complaints from individuals that their rights have been infringed upon by the government. Five of the human rights treaty bodies (CCPR, CERD, CAT, CEDAW and CRPD) may, under particular circumstances (specific details can be found at www.ohchr.org), consider individual complaints or communications from individuals. The Convention on Migrant Workers also contains provision for allowing individual communications to be considered by the

CMW; these provisions will become operative when ten states parties have made the necessary declaration under article 77.

The committee's opinions or 'views' in relation to individual complaints are not the same as the judgements of international or domestic courts. Although they may pronounce on the compatibility of government actions with treaty obligations, their opinions are not enforceable in any legal sense. However, their persuasive force is often such that the government concerned may be inclined to adjust its laws or policies accordingly as can be seen in the examples considered later in this chapter.

The OHCHR also has a regional structure and in some cases also a country presence. Regional offices and centres are established on the basis of a standard agreement between OHCHR and the host country, following consultations with countries within the same region (OHCHR 2009b). Regional offices and centres focus on cross-cutting regional human rights concerns and also support, at national level, follow-up to treaty bodies and special procedures as well as matters relating to the Universal Periodic Review (UPR), discussed later. Regional offices and centres work closely with regional and subregional intergovernmental organisations, including to provide support on institutional and thematic issues.

The activities, analyses, conclusions and recommendations of regional bodies are reported to the High Commissioner including through her annual report to the Human Rights Council. At the end of 2010, OHCHR had twelve regional offices/centres: in East Africa (Addis Ababa), Southern Africa (Pretoria), West Africa (Dakar), Central Africa (Yaoundé), South-East Asia (Bangkok), the Pacific (Suva), the Middle East (Beirut), Central Asia (Bishkek), Europe (Brussels), Central America (Panama City), South America (Santiago de Chile), and South-West Asia and the Arab Region (Doha) (OHCHR 2011a).

Human Rights Council

The Human Rights Council was established by the UN General Assembly in March 2006, as a successor to the Commission on Human Rights. The Human Rights Council is an intergovernmental body within the UN system. It is made up of representatives from forty-seven countries, and is responsible for strengthening the promotion and protection of human rights around the globe. One year after holding its first meeting, on 18 June 2007, the Council adopted its 'Institution-building package', providing direction for its future work. As a result of this, a Universal Periodic Review mechanism was set up (see below). Other features included a new Advisory Committee which serves as the Council's 'think tank', providing it with expertise and advice on thematic human rights issues and the revised 'Complaints Procedure' mechanism which allows individuals and organisations to bring complaints about human rights violations to the attention of the Council. The Human Rights Council also continues to work closely with the UN Special Procedures established by the former Commission on Human Rights and now assumed by the Council. These are discussed further below.

Universal Periodic Review

The Universal Periodic Review (UPR) is a unique process which involves a review of the human rights records of all UN member states once every four years. The UPR is a state-driven process, under the auspices of the Human Rights Council, which provides the opportunity for each state to declare what actions they have taken to improve the human rights situations in their countries and to fulfil their human rights obligations. The UPR is designed to ensure equal treatment for every country when their human rights situations are assessed. The UPR was created through the UN General Assembly on 15 March 2006 by resolution 60/251, which established the Human Rights Council itself. It is a cooperative process which, on 13 October 2011, completed its first cycle, having reviewed the human rights records of every country. Currently, no other universal mechanism of this kind exists. The ultimate aim of this mechanism is to improve the human rights situation in all countries and address human rights violations wherever they occur.

The reviews are based on information provided by three sources: a report by the state under review; a compendium of information contained in the reports of independent human rights experts and groups, known as the Special Procedures, human rights treaty bodies, and other UN entities; a compendium of information from other stakeholders including non-governmental organisations and national human rights institutions. NGOs can play a significant role in the process as Moss (2010) describes. NGO submissions are published on the OHCHR website for the state concerned and thus become a part of a central reference on the human rights situation for the country concerned. This provides a valuable opportunity for advocacy. NGO reports can include specific recommendations, which may then be picked up in the review sessions. Moss analysed the proceedings of the second session of the UPR in which sixteen states were reviewed. He finds that a total of 745 factual statements, observations or recommendations by NGOs were included in the summaries of 'other stakeholder information' used in the second session. Of these 523 (or 70 per cent) correspond to recommendations made by member states to the states under review, and 199 of those were accepted by the relevant state under review (Moss 2010). Moss's analysis further suggests that forming a broad national coalition of NGOs for advocacy around the UPR process can be particularly effective.

Special procedures

'Special procedures' is the general name given to the mechanisms established by the Human Rights Council to address either specific country situations or thematic issues in all parts of the world. At the end of 2010, there were thirty-three thematic and eight country mandates (OHCHR 2011b), with fifty-five individual experts who were mandate-holders. The Office of the High Commissioner for Human Rights provides these mechanisms with personnel, policy, research and logistical support for the discharge of their mandates. The mandate-holders report and advise on human rights from a thematic or country-specific perspective. The aim is that their independence, impartiality and flexibility enable the Special Procedures to play a critical role in promoting and protecting human rights. The experts deal with situations wherever they may occur in the world, including in the context of crises and emergencies.

With the support of the Office of the United Nations High Commissioner for Human Rights (OHCHR), mandate-holders discharge their responsibilities in a number of different ways. First, they undertake country visits (fact-finding missions). Secondly, they act on individual cases and concerns of a broader, structural nature by sending communications to states in which they bring alleged violations to their attention. Thirdly, they can conduct thematic studies and convene expert consultations, develop international human rights standards, engage in advocacy, raise public awareness, and provide advice and support for technical cooperation. Special Procedures report annually to the Human Rights Council; the majority of the mandates also report to the General Assembly.

Mandate-holders are referred to as independent experts or special rapporteurs; they serve in a personal capacity, are not UN staff members and do not receive financial remuneration. Countries that currently have a country mandate are Burundi, Cambodia, Democratic People's Republic of Korea, Haiti, Myanmar, Palestinian territories occupied since 1967, Somalia and Sudan (OHCHR 2011b). Thematic mandates include special rapporteurs on: the right of everyone to the enjoyment of the highest attainable standard of physical and mental health (since 2002); the sale of children, child prostitution and child pornography (since 1990), violence against women (since 1994); the situation of human rights and fundamental freedoms of indigenous peoples (since 2001); and trafficking in persons, especially women and children (since 2004).

Holding governments to account

As has been made clear above, the UN system relies, to a great extent, on powers of persuasion, or, as some have put it 'naming and shaming', to encourage governments to change laws, policy or practice in the direction necessary to promote, protect or fulfil rights. This section considers two contrasting examples of reactions of one country, Australia, to adverse communications from monitoring committees.

An example of where the UN system helped to effect positive change is the adverse opinion of the Human Rights Committee (as the monitoring committee for the ICCPR is called) in the Toonen case concerning the criminal laws relating to homosexuality in Tasmania. This resulted from a communication made by an individual, Toonen, arguing that the laws violated his rights as a homosexual man. The challenged provisions of the Tasmanian legislation were said to violate the articles of the ICCPR in three respects. The first of these was that the legislation made no distinction between sexual activity in public and in private and thus brought private activity into the public domain. Second, the legislation distinguished between individuals in the exercise of their right to privacy on the basis of sexual activity, sexual orientation and sexual identity, thus discriminating in its effects. Third, the legislation did not outlaw homosexual activity between consenting homosexual women in private and outlawed only some forms of consenting heterosexual activity between adult men and women in private, again showing discrimination.

Toonen's communication was lodged in 1991, and the Committee reported its views in 1994 (United Nations Human Rights Committee Views on Communication, 488/1992, adopted 31 March 1994). Australia summarised its response to this in its third report to the Human Rights Committee (CCPR/C/AUS/98/3: 4–5, paras 12–14), where it reported that:

> Communication 488/1992 N. Toonen v. Australia
>
> 12. Sections 122 (a) and (c) and 123 of the 1924 Criminal Code of Tasmania made homosexual sexual activity a criminal offence in Tasmania. The author of communication 488/1992 alleged that these provisions were discriminatory under the terms of articles 2.1, 17 and 26 of the Covenant.
>
> 13. The Human Rights Committee declared the communication admissible on 5 November 1992 and published its final views on 31 March 1994. It found that sections 122 (a) and (c) and 123 of the Tasmanian code were an arbitrary interference with privacy and placed Australia in breach of article 17.
>
> 14. In response to the Committee's views, the Federal Attorney-General held discussions with the Tasmanian Premier and Attorney-General. The Tasmanian Government's position was that no action would be taken in response to the Committee's findings. Accordingly, the Federal Government introduced legislation to provide protection for all Australians from arbitrary interferences with sexual privacy. The legislation, entitled the Human Rights (Sexual Conduct) Act, came into force on 19 December 1994. For further details on the Act, the Committee is referred to the commentary on article 17 below.

This laid the basis for further challenge to the Tasmanian criminal code, this time in the Australian High Court. Eventually, in 1998 Tasmanian Anti-Discrimination Act passed into law, hailed by Croome (quoted in Bernardi 2001) as 'one of the best pieces of anti-discrimination legislation in the country'. A full discussion of the case can be found in Editors (1994) and Bernardi (2001). In July 2011, Navi Pillay, the current UN High Commissioner of Human Rights, released a video looking back at the case which she describes as 'a watershed with wide-ranging implications for the human rights of millions of people'. She continues:

> Since 1994, more than 30 countries have taken steps to abolish the offence of homosexuality ... Some have enacted new laws providing greater protection against discrimination on grounds of sexual orientation or gender identity. ... And in many parts of the world, we have witnessed a remarkable shift in public attitudes, in favour of greater acceptance of gay and lesbian people.

Nick Toonen says he was proud to have been involved in such an important moment in the advancement of human rights:

It's humbling that so many people around the world have benefitted from the decision in my case ...The obvious message from the case was that gay rights are human rights, but equally important was the message that everyday people like me can take effective action to protect human rights. My case was very much a group effort and I want to acknowledge everyone who fought for gay law reform in Tasmania as well as the many gay, lesbian, bisexual and transgender people around the world who continue to fight for their rights and their lives.

In the video, Ms Pillay says the Human Rights Committee's decision in the Toonen case had made clear that the right to be free from discrimination applies to everyone: gay, straight, lesbian or bisexual. She says the result 'reverberated around the world' when Toonen's complaint was upheld. The Human Rights Committee has since reaffirmed its position in successive cases, entrenching in human rights law the principle that no country is entitled to discriminate against people on grounds of their sexuality. But, as the High Commissioner reports, criminal sanctions remain in place in more than seventy countries, exposing millions to the risk of arrest, imprisonment, even in some cases the death penalty: 'Not because they have harmed anyone else or pose a threat to others, but simply for being who they are and for loving another human being' (all quotes from the Press Release that accompanied the release of the video, www.humanrights.gov.au/about/media/news/2011/62_11.html, 28 July 2011).

A contrasting example is provided by the case (*A v Australia*) concerning the detention of asylum seekers which demonstrates that, ultimately, however, if a state should decide that it does not wish to 'implement' the decision of a committee, then it can do so with relative impunity. This was the case with Australia's reaction to the adverse opinion of the Human Rights Committee issued in 1997 in the so-called Boat-People case (*A v Australia*) concerning the detention of asylum seekers and their treatment in detention. No action has been taken by the Australian Government, nor is any planned, to address the concerns raised by the Committee, and the question of the detention of asylum seekers continues to be controversial to the present day. A full report on the case is found in UN document CCPR/C/59/D/560/1993.

NGOs in the global system

As has already been seen, NGOs can play a particularly important part in raising issues within the global system, and there are a number of very significant globally based NGOs who are key stakeholders in the global system. In this section, a brief overview of some of the most significant is given. Table 2.6 gives details of the web addresses of these organisations, which provide extensive detail on the organisations and their current campaigns, and give access to annual reports and other publications and resources. Many of these organisations make full use of social media to support their advocacy and other efforts.

The genesis of Amnesty International lay in an article by a British lawyer, Peter Benenson, published in the *Observer* newspaper, on 28 May 1961. 'The Forgotten

Table 2.6 Selected NGOs in the global system

General NGOs	
Amnesty International	http://www.amnesty.org website available in English, Arabic, French and Spanish
Human Rights Watch	http://www.hrw.org website available in English, Arabic, French, Spanish, Chinese, Russian, German, Hebrew and Japanese; plus limited information in other languages
International Network for Economic, Social and Cultural Rights (ESCR-Net)	http://www.escr-net.org/
International Service for Human Rights	http://www.ishr.ch/
Commonwealth Human Rights Initiative (CHRI)	http://www.humanrightsinitiative.org/
Health specific NGOs	
Center for Reproductive Rights	http://www.reproductiverights.org
People's Health Movement (PHM)	http://www.phmovement.org/
Médecins Sans Frontières (MSF)	http://www.msf.org/ most relevant for its Campaign on Access to Essential Medicines now on a separate website: http://www.msfaccess.org/
Stop Torture in Health Care	http://www.stoptortureinhealthcare.org/
Women's Global Network for Reproductive Rights	http://www.wgnrr.org/
Profession specific NGOs	
Physicians for Human Rights	http://physiciansforhumanrights.org/
Global Lawyers and Physicians (GLP)	http://www.globallawyersandphysicians.org/

Prisoners' was written after he read about two Portuguese students who had been imprisoned for raising their wine glasses in a toast to freedom, and he launched the 'Appeal for Amnesty 1961'. A first international meeting was held in July 1961, with delegates from Belgium, the UK, France, Germany, Ireland, Switzerland and the USA, at which it was decided to establish 'a permanent international movement in defence of freedom of opinion and religion'. The following year Amnesty International groups were started in Australia, Belgium, Denmark, Greece, Ireland, Norway, Sweden and the USA. At a conference in Belgium, the groups decided to set up a permanent organisation to be known as 'Amnesty International'. By 2011, when Amnesty International celebrated its fiftieth anniversary, it had grown into a global movement of more than 3 million supporters, members and activists in more than 150 countries and territories who campaign to end grave abuses of human rights. Amnesty's vision is 'for every person to enjoy all the rights enshrined in the Universal Declaration of Human Rights and other international human rights standards'. The organisation is independent of any government, political ideology, economic interest or religion and is funded mainly by membership and public donations.

Human Rights Watch began in 1978 and is one of the world's leading independent organisations dedicated to defending and protecting human rights. It is an independent, non-governmental organisation, supported by contributions from private individuals and foundations worldwide. It accepts no government funds, directly or indirectly. A case study presents a recent example of the work of Human Rights Watch (p. 30).

The International Network for Economic, Social and Cultural Rights (ESCR-Net) was designed as a decentralised structure that complements and strengthens, rather than replicates, the efforts of organisations working at the national or grassroots level by allowing them to build bridges across regions, disciplines and approaches. As an international human rights network, ESCR-Net has not incorporated as an NGO or sought independent non-profit status in any particular country. For the operations of its Secretariat, currently based in New York City, ESCR-Net became a project of the Tides Center (www.tidescenter.org), a non-profit public charity exempt from federal income tax under Sections 501(c)3 and 509(a)1 of the Internal Revenue Code, in September 2004.

The substantive work of ESCR-Net is carried out through decentralised structures that are comprised of and coordinated by members based in different countries. These structures can take the form of a Working Group, Initiative or Discussion Group, each providing a different way for organisations to work together on an issue of shared concern and enable joint action. ESCR-Net seeks to strengthen economic, social and cultural rights by working with organisations and activists worldwide to facilitate mutual learning and strategy exchange; develop new tools and resources; engage in advocacy; and provide information-sharing and networking.

The International Service for Human Rights (ISHR) is an international non-governmental organisation based in Geneva, at the heart of the United Nations human rights system, with a small branch office in New York. The ISHR was created in 1984 with the objective of bridging the gap between the UN human rights system and the realities of the work of human rights defenders at the national level. It has enabled defenders to access the UN system and to effectively participate at the international level. Over time, ISHR's geographic reach has broadened to incorporate regional systems of protection. Beginning with a staff of three in Geneva, ISHR grew to include an office in New York and currently counts a total of fifteen expert staff. While its capacity has increased at all levels, advocacy, training and information services have remained at the heart of ISHR's work since the beginning, with work at national, regional and international levels.

Finally, in terms of generalist human rights international NGOs, there is the Commonwealth Human Rights Initiative (CHRI), which is an independent, non-partisan, international non-governmental organisation, mandated to ensure the practical realisation of human rights in the countries of the Commonwealth. In 1987, several Commonwealth associations founded CHRI because they felt that,

Case study: Protecting the rights of LGBT people: NGO advocacy in action

In response to a global advocacy campaign led by Human Rights Watch, the UN General Assembly held a rare revote on a resolution protecting people from extrajudicial killings.

The provision on sexual orientation was first added to the UN resolution on extrajudicial killings in 1999 at the insistence of the UN Special Rapporteur on Torture, whose findings evidenced the link between homophobia, perceived sexual orientation and fatal hate crimes in a number of places around the world. During a November 2010 meeting of the UN committee that oversees decisions on human rights, that part of the resolution was removed. The initiative for the provision's removal was spearheaded, ostensibly for religious and cultural reasons, by some members of the Organisation of the Islamic Conference and of the United Nation's African Regional Group, including Uganda, South Africa, and Rwanda.

Human Rights Watch took a number of significant steps:

- Boris Dittrich, Human Rights Watch's LGBT rights advocacy director, used a UN event he was co-organising to celebrate International Human Rights Day on 10 December as a catalyst to prompt a revote. UN Secretary-General Ban Ki-moon and US Ambassador to the United Nations Susan Rice were invited, and both accepted. The Secretary-General opened the session by calling for an end to laws that criminalise consenting homosexual conduct. Rice, during her keynote speech, announced that the United States sought to reopen the debate on the controversial amendment at a meeting of the UN General Assembly just eleven days later.
- Human Rights Watch's South Africa director, Sipho Mthathi, increased pressure on the government in Pretoria, and encouraged South African LGBT rights groups to do the same. This was supported by Dittrich's appearance on South African television pointing out the contrast between the robust protections for the LGBT community in the South African constitution, and a vote in favour of an amendment that would remove protections for LGBT people.
- HRW contacted as many diplomats ahead of the reopened debate as possible. This outreach helped secure fresh support from many countries, including a block of seven countries in the Caribbean Community (Caricom). Meetings were held with UN mission diplomats from Colombia and Suriname, and LGBT human rights activists in these countries mobilised. Both of these countries changed their vote, as did South Africa.
- During the final vote by the General Assembly, the UN Ambassador from Rwanda made a strong statement in favour of undoing the homophobic

> amendment. Together with cooperation from Argentina, Belgium, Brazil, France, the Netherlands, Norway and Gabon, these efforts led to an overwhelming majority of ninety-four countries in favour of restoring the resolution to ensure that LGBT people would continue to be protected.
>
> (Extracted from www.hrw.org/en/news/2011/02/14/restoring-protection-lgbt-people-against-extrajudicial-executions, accessed May 2011)

while the member countries had both a common set of values and legal principles from which to work and a forum within which to promote human rights, there was relatively little focus on human rights issues. CHRI has its headquarters in New Delhi, India, and offices in London, UK, and Accra, Ghana; it is particularly active in India.

In terms of human rights issues most directly connected to health, there are a number of different NGOs. The People's Health Movement (PHM) developed as a response to the failure of the goal of 'Health for All by the Year 2000' in the Alma Ata declaration to be realised. By the end of the year 2000 several international organisations, civil society movements, NGOs and women's groups organised the first People's Health Assembly in December 2000 in Savar, Bangladesh. Here they formulated and endorsed the People's Charter for Health. The PHM rose from this Assembly as a body of health rights proponents who would demand Health for All Now across the globe, a worldwide citizens' movement committed to making the Alma Ata dream a reality. PHM is considered in more detail in Chapters 6 and 12.

Médecins Sans Frontières (MSF) is an international medical humanitarian organisation created by doctors and journalists in France in 1971. It provides emergency medical assistance to populations in danger in more than sixty countries, delivering emergency aid to people affected by armed conflict, epidemics, health care exclusion and natural or man-made disasters. It also set up the Campaign for Access to Essential Medicines in 1999 to push for access to, and the development of, life-saving and life-prolonging medicines, diagnostic tests and vaccines for patients in MSF programmes and beyond.

The Center for Reproductive Rights, based in New York, is a global legal advocacy organisation dedicated to reproductive rights, with expertise in both US constitutional and international human rights law. Their cases before national courts, United Nations committees and regional human rights bodies have expanded access to reproductive health care, including birth control, safe abortion, prenatal and obstetric care, and unbiased information. Some of their work is discussed further later in the book.

Women's Global Network for Reproductive Rights (WGNRR) is a southern-based global network that builds and strengthens movements for sexual and reproductive health, rights and justice. WGNRR works to realise the full sexual and reproductive health and rights of all people, with a particular focus on the most marginalised. They argue that achieving this goal requires transformative social change. Since 2009, the Organisation's Coordination Office operates completely from Manila in the Philippines, based in the global south. WGNRR has collaborated with the People's Health Movement (PHM) under the broad umbrella campaign of Women's Access to Health.

Most recently there is 'Stop Torture in Health Care', a campaign launched in 2011 by the Open Society Foundations (based in the US). Three topics make up the bulk of their work: forced sterilisation; denial of pain relief; and detention as treatment.

Finally, some NGOs are profession-specific. Physicians for Human Rights is an independent organisation that was founded in 1986 on the idea that health professionals, with their specialised skills, ethical duties and credible voices, are uniquely positioned to stop human rights violations. They use their investigations and expertise to advocate for the: prevention of individual or small-scale acts of violence from becoming mass atrocities; protection of internationally guaranteed rights of individuals and civilian populations; and prosecution of those who violate human rights. Physicians for Human Rights is based in Cambridge, Massachusetts, with an office in Washington, DC. Global Lawyers and Physicians (GLP) is a non-profit, non-governmental organisation that focuses on health and human rights issues. GLP was founded in 1996 at an international symposium on health at the United States Holocaust Memorial Museum to commemorate the fiftieth anniversary of the Nuremberg Doctors Trial on the premise that physicians and lawyers, working together transnationally, can be a much more effective force for human rights than either profession can working separately.

Ongoing debates, ongoing development

It is often argued that rights are culturally independent, as for example in the quote from Boutros Boutros Ghali that begun this chapter. Not all agree however. Some argue that the concept of universality is culturally constructed. Human rights are viewed as representing the particular belief systems of some cultures and societies rather than those of all cultures and societies. This is the so-called cultural relativist argument, the very rationale of which is to deny claims of universality. Accordingly, in their modern form, human rights are considered a Western construct of limited application to non-Western nations. Some Asian political leaders have adopted this cultural relativist argument; see for example, Kausikan (1996). Katsumata (2009), on the other hand, argues that within ASEAN countries have been adopting the norm of human rights, and sees this in part as recognition of the compatibility of human rights with Asian cultures and values, a view reinforced by Levinson's chronology (2003). Meijknecht and De Vries's analysis (2010) however identifies a number of areas in the treatment of minorities and indigenous peoples where appeals to 'Asian values' seem to de-prioritise human rights in favour of other goals such as economic development. Manea (2009) offers a historical analysis of the dynamics of interaction both within ASEAN and in relation to the UN and EU, exploring how this has resulted in a series of shifts in ASEAN self-conception of its regional identity and its stance on human rights. Space precludes a detailed treatment here, especially as the debate is extremely wide-ranging. See for example: Nagengast's careful discussion (1997) of debates in relation to women, minorities and indigenous peoples; Durrant (2008) who focuses on the issue of physical punishment of children in relation to culture and the rights of children; and finally Bickenbach (2009) who examines the Convention on the Rights of Persons with Disabilities in relation to therapeutic strategies of respecting cultural differences. For an invigorating and critical examination of the arguments on cultural relativism in general, see Tilley (2000). In terms of the historical period around the creation of the UN, Bhagavan (2010) challenges some of the existing interpretations of this period by exploring the significant role that the newly independent India played, particularly in the creation of the UDHR.

A further example of both the influence of culture and the need for ongoing development of our understandings of human rights is provided by Goldingay (2007, 2009) in her research on young female prisoners in New Zealand, who problematises the notion of 'best interests' as it is written in the Convention on the Rights of the Child, which is often taken as supporting separate facilities for young prisoners. For young Maori female prisoners in New Zealand in a non-age-separated prison for women, her informants reported that, for a number of reasons, ongoing close relationships with adults were essential for their wellbeing (Goldingay 2007). Her larger study (Goldingay 2009) illustrates how for Maori and Pacific Islander cultures, the notion of 'best interests' of the child may not align well with separation into age-specific facilities, which may deny young people access to their culture, with negative consequences for health and wellbeing. Her findings certainly point to the need to consider cultural factors carefully in interpreting 'best interests'.

Another area of debate is the notion of intergenerational rights, in two senses: first, in terms of the responsibility for action by present generations to provide redress for past human rights violations, and second, in terms of consideration of the rights of future generations. As relevant examples of the first of these, the Canadian government has provided significant funds for the Canadian Aboriginal Healing Foundation in reparation for the human rights violations of Canadian indigenous peoples in the residential school system, as well as compensation payments to individual survivors (Castellano *et al.* 2008). In Australia, although an important symbolic apology was delivered on 13 February 2008 by the then Prime Minister Kevin Rudd to the stolen generations of indigenous children who were forcibly removed from their families (http://australia.gov.au/about-australia/our-country/our-people/apology-to-australias-indigenous-peoples), debate continues about whether monetary compensation should also be provided, as the original report of the national inquiry recommended (Bringing Them Home 1997). Turning to the rights of future generations, this has particular relevance for those within the environmental movements, where the argument is that there is a moral obligation to respect and protect the rights of future generations in the context provided not only by environmental pollution, but by the increasing evidence of the likely adverse affects of climate change (e.g. see Zarsky 2002).

Fulfilling human rights is a *necessary prerequisite* for health of individuals and populations. In the wake of globalisation and privatisation, increasing attention must be paid to the role of non-state actors because they are influencing the health and wellbeing of people to an unprecedented extent – comparable to (or even greater than) the influence of governments (OHCHR 2000). Amongst other things, this calls for a need to reinforce the commitment and capacity of governments to ensure that actions taken by the private sector, as well as other actors, are informed by and comply with human rights principles. Current structures are generally insufficient for NGOs or governments to monitor effectively and hold corporations operating on a national scale accountable; the problem is compounded for multinationals, who may escape accountability within states, and for whom there is no international human rights law that applies directly to them or their actions. Chapter 3 explores this issue further.

There is also ongoing debate about the development of the global system itself. The High Commissioner for Human Rights since 2008, Navi Pillay, has initiated a consultation on strengthening the UN system, and is pushing for continued efforts to mainstream human rights in all UN operations, an increased budget to reflect the increased volume of work that the OHCHR undertakes, and is placing increased emphasis on strengthening the role of National Human Rights Institutions (NHRIs), NGOs and on human rights education (OHCHR 2009b).

3 Regional human rights systems

In this chapter the focus of attention shifts to examine the various regional systems. These exist in a number of different senses: first, in terms of systems linking a group of countries or member states, and second in terms of systems linking different national human rights institutions. There are also regionally based NGOs of various types, and global NGOs often have a regional structure to their operations. The OHCHR also presides over a regional system. This covers the whole globe, however, it does not exactly align with the regional systems discussed in this chapter. There is considerable variation in these systems, both in terms of their operation and the extent to which they can exert direct influence on the states within their boundaries. Established regional human rights systems, based on a human rights charter, together with some regional enforcement mechanisms, exist in Africa, the Americas and Europe and these are considered in separate sections below. In Asia and the Middle East, more limited regional developments have taken place, and sections below consider each of these in turn.

It is obviously impossible in a single chapter to include a comprehensive review of the achievements of each of the regional systems, especially as there is only limited research available. Instead the aim has been to incorporate throughout the chapter different examples of the operation and effectiveness of systems. These have been selected to illustrate the potential impact of such systems in tackling health inequity and increasing social justice, while also identifying some of the challenges and difficulties that remain. Table 3.1 presents some key features of the regional human rights systems, summarising their origins, membership and organisation.

Africa

The basic regional human rights instrument for Africa is the African Charter on Human and Peoples' Rights, this is also known as the Banjul Charter, after the place where it was drafted, the city of Banjul in the Gambia. The Charter was adopted in June 1981 by the Assembly of Heads of State and Government of the Organization of African Unity (the Organization of African Unity was replaced by the African Union in 2000). The Charter came into force in October 1986.

Human and Peoples' Rights are set out in articles 1 to 26 of the Charter. It is worth noting the particular formulation used in the Charter, as well as within the title

Table 3.1 Summary features of regional human rights systems

	Origins	Membership	Organization/operation
Africa	1981 – African Charter on Human and Peoples' Rights (Banjul Charter)	Charter applies to the 53 states who are members of the African Union. 25 African States have acknowledged the Court's jurisdiction	Through two bodies: African Commission on Human and Peoples' Rights based in Banjul, Gambia and African Court on Human and Peoples' Rights, Arusha, Tanzania. Individuals may raise complaints.
Americas	1948 – American Declaration of the rights and duties of man 1969 – American Convention on Human Rights Plus other protocols and conventions	22 American States recognise jurisdiction of the court (a further 2 have ratified the Convention only)	Through two bodies: Inter-American Commission on Human Rights (IACHR) based in Washington, D.C. and Inter-American Court of Human Rights, San José, Costa Rica. Individuals may petition the Commission
Asia	1967 – Association of Southeast Asian Nations (ASEAN) established	10 member States	ASEAN Intergovernmental Commission on Human Rights (AICHR) set up in 2009. Still not clear whether AICHR will receive complaints from individuals. Rules of procedure yet to be established
Europe – 1	1950 – European Convention on Human Rights, entered into force 1953	Council of Europe members, currently 47	Through European Court of Human Rights. Individuals can take cases there. Can direct changes in country law
Europe – 2	2000 – Charter of Fundamental Rights of the European Union	EU member states	Originally, 'Soft' law – rules of conduct that have no legally binding force*, powers strengthened in 2009
Middle East	1968 – Council of the League of Arab States founded the Permanent Arab Commission on Human Rights (PACHR)	22 member states	Modernised version of Arab charter on Human Rights came into force in 2008. PACHR works mainly around rights of Arabs living in Israeli-occupied territories
Organisation of the Islamic Conference (OIC)	1969 – OIC established, present Charter adopted 2008, 1990 – Cairo Declaration on Human Rights in Islam 2004 – Covenant on the rights of the child in Islam	57 member states across four continents	No reporting or monitoring mechanisms exist

*definition from Trubeck and Trubeck (2005)

of the Commission and Court, with reference to 'human and peoples' rights' rather than simply 'human rights'; this can be seen as a move to explicitly include the notion of 'collective rights' held by a group as well as 'individual rights' held by every person. Article 16 in the Charter makes an explicit statement on the right to health: '1. Every individual shall have the right to enjoy the best attainable state of physical and mental health. 2. State Parties to the present Charter shall take the necessary measures to protect the health of their people and to ensure that they receive medical attention when they are sick.' Health is also referred to in items 1 and 4 of article 18 which read respectively: 'the family shall be the natural unit and basis of society. It shall be protected by the State which shall take care of its physical health and moral needs' and 'The aged and the disabled shall also have the right to special measures of protection in keeping with their physical or moral needs'. Other articles in the Charter relate closely to the social determinants of health, in particular the right to work (article 15), the right to education (article 17), use of wealth and natural resources (article 21) and the provision of environment favourable to development (article 24).

In the case of article 21, clauses recognise the deleterious effects that foreign exploitation, in particular by 'international monopolies', has had, and makes provision for compensation and recovery. The final clauses in this article, clauses 4 and 5, state:

> 4. State Parties to the present Charter shall individually and collectively exercise the right to free disposal of their wealth and natural resources with a view to strengthening African Unity and solidarity.
>
> 5. State Parties to the present Charter shall undertake to eliminate all forms of foreign exploitation particularly that practised by international monopolies so as to enable their peoples to fully benefit from the advantages derived from their national resources.

Acting on these clauses in practice has proved challenging, as a later case study on the Niger Delta region shows.

African Commission on Human and Peoples' Rights

The Commission was established by article 30 of the Banjul Charter. The Commission is composed of eleven members elected by secret ballot by the Assembly of Heads of State and Government for a six-year renewable term. The Commissioners elect two of their members as Chairperson and Vice-Chairperson for a two-year renewable period; the Secretary to the Commission is appointed by the Chairperson of the African Union Commission. The members serve in their personal and individual capacity and have full independence in the discharge of their duties and diplomatic privileges and immunities. They are supported by a Secretariat provided by the Organization for African Unity, later African Union.

The functions of the Commission are set out in article 45 of the Banjul Charter and can be summarised as the protection and promotion of rights and the interpretation of the provisions of the Charter, together with the production of principles and rules to assist in solving legal problems relating to rights and fundamental freedoms. The Commission is able to investigate and research relevant issues, and also can organise a wide range of meetings, symposia, etc. in discharge of its functions. The Commission can receive communications from individuals as well as states. There is a requirement that local remedies, if they exist, must have been exhausted first, unless it is deemed that such local procedures are unduly prolonged. On receipt of communications from individuals or organisations (other than states), the Commissioners vote on whether the communication should be considered, the decision being with the majority. Once it is decided that a communication is to be considered, the relevant state concerned is notified and, if after deliberation it appears that there are serious or massive violations of rights involved, the Commission will report this to the Assembly of Heads of State and Government who may request the Commission to undertake an in-depth study; in cases of emergency the Chairperson of the Assembly may request a study.

As at 20 April 2011, 187 decisions in relation to 247 communications are documented on the Commission's website, covering the period 1988 to 2009. They relate to forty-one of the fifty-three countries in the African Union. The two articles most closely connected to the right to health (articles 16 and 18) are involved in eleven of these decisions (resulting from fifty-one communications), which involve thirteen countries. Except for two cases where the communication was withdrawn by the complainant, all cases were found proven. The majority of the communications related to the consequences of armed conflict within or between states and arrest, detention and torture; some involve systematic discrimination against particular national or ethnic groups. In two cases, there are direct consequences for health systems and public health, and these are described in the two case studies.

African Court on Human and Peoples' Rights

The African Court on Human and Peoples' Rights was established by a Protocol to the African Charter on Human and Peoples' Rights. This Protocol was adopted by member states of the then Organization of African Unity in Ouagadougou, Burkina Faso, in June 1998, and entered into force in January 2004. The Court started its operations in Addis Ababa, Ethiopia, in November 2006 and moved to its permanent seat in Arusha, Tanzania, in August 2007.

Submissions to the Court can be made by the African Commission on Human Rights, by states, by African Intergovernmental Organisations or by individuals or NGOs. Thus far (up to September 2011) only six cases are reported on the Court's website, five of which deal with postponements or judgment regarding lack of jurisdiction and referral to the ACHPR, one, December 2009, reports on a submission by an individual against the state of Senegal, which was judged inadmissible (discussed in Mujuzi 2010). The sixth case, brought by the African Commission on Human and Peoples' Rights against the state of Libya, dated 25 March 2011, ordered provisional measures, requesting that Libya refrain from 'any

Case study: The rights of the Ogoni people in the Niger Delta region

In 1996, the Social and Economic Rights Action Center and the Center for Economic and Social Rights in Nigeria lodged a communication in respect of the actions of the government of Nigeria in collaboration with the Shell Petroleum Development Corporation. Their communication alleged that the oil operations in the Niger Delta region were causing environmental degradation and health problems for the Ogoni people as a result of environmental contamination. There were further charges regarding the direct involvement of the military in attacking, burning and destroying Ogoni villages and homes under false pretexts. The Commission's decision found the government in violation of multiple articles of the Charter (ACHPR 2001) and appealed to the government to ensure protection of the environment, health and livelihood of the Ogoni people, supporting this with a number of specific recommendations. Nigeria's latest periodic country report on the implementation of the African Charter on Human and Peoples' Rights, covering 2005–8 (Federal Ministry of Justice 2008), describes a variety of measures put in place to address the problems, including the creation of a new ministry of the Niger Delta with a view to ensuring effective implementation of a comprehensive master plan, programmes and direct intervention projects in the region. In the Commission's set of concluding observations and recommendations on this report (ACHPR 2008), concern is expressed about the lack of change in the operations of transnational corporations in the Niger Delta, affecting the rights to food, shelter and the environment of the people in the region, and a lack of effective government monitoring mechanisms, and there is a specific recommendation on the creation of these. Recent research documents the involvement of Shell, through payments to groups linked to violence, in cases of serious violence and human rights abuses in the Delta region from 2000 to 2010 (Amunwa 2011). Finally, UNEP (2011) provides a comprehensive environmental assessment and summarises the public health impacts of the degradation, in particular arising from water contamination, making comprehensive recommendations for environmental restoration including at the regulatory, operational and monitoring levels.

action that would result in loss of life or violation of physical integrity of persons' (African Court on Human and Peoples' Rights 2011: 7).

In July 2008, the African Union made the decision to merge the Court with the African Court of Justice (established through the Constitutive Act of the African Union) to create a single African Court of Justice and Human Rights. This will not however come into force until ratification of the relevant Protocol by fifteen African states; as at 20 April 2011, only three states had ratified this protocol.

> **Case study: Mental health services in the Gambia**
>
> The government of the Gambia was summoned by the African Commission on Human and Peoples' Rights for alleged violations of human rights of people suffering from mental disorders detained in the country's only mental health facility, the Campama Psychiatric Unit. The case was brought by two mental health advocates (communication 241/01). The Commission's decision, reported in May 2003 (ACHPR 2003), found the Gambia in violation of the human rights of inpatients and made specific recommendations on the need for legal reform and changes in the health care system. Following that decision, the Republic of the Gambia embarked on an exercise to address mental health service delivery within the country and in November 2004 requested technical assistance from WHO in developing a draft mental health policy and plan (WHO 2007a); WHO responded by providing the national drafting committee with relevant technical guidance material, access to additional resources and support through providing comments on drafts. A National Mental Health Policy and Strategic Plan was finalised in 2007 and implementation is under way (AFRO 2009). However, the Gambia has not submitted a regular report to the Commission since the decision in 2010, and reform of legislation has not yet occurred.

Americas

The regional system in the Americas is based in the Organization of American States (OAS). The First International Conference of American States was held in Washington, DC, October 1889 to April 1890; however the Charter governing the present-day operation of the OAS did not come into force until 1970. There are two bodies responsible for the promotion and protection of human rights in the Inter-American System, the Inter-American Commission on Human Rights (IACHR) and the Inter-American Court of Human Rights.

The Inter-American Commission on Human Rights is an organ of the OAS and is based in Washington, DC. Its mandate derives from the OAS Charter, OAS Declaration of the Rights and Duties of Man (with content broadly similar to the UDHR), the American Convention on Human Rights and the Commission's Statute. The IACHR consists of seven members who carry out their functions independently, without representing any particular country. Its members are elected by the General Assembly of the OAS for a period of four years and they may be re-elected only once. The Executive Secretariat carries out the tasks delegated to it by the IACHR and provides the Commission with legal and administrative support in its pursuit of its functions. The IACHR was created in 1959, and held its first meeting in 1960 (IACHR 2011). Since 1961, it has carried out visits to countries to produce country reports and reports on particular topics, and since 1965 it has heard individual petitions regarding alleged human rights violations (IACHR 2011).

The American Convention on Human Rights ('the American Convention') was adopted in 1969 and came into force in 1978. As of December 2010, a total of twenty-four member states were parties to the Convention: Argentina, Barbados, Bolivia, Brazil, Chile, Colombia, Costa Rica, Dominica, the Dominican Republic, Ecuador, El Salvador, Grenada, Guatemala, Haiti, Honduras, Jamaica, Mexico, Nicaragua, Panama, Paraguay, Peru, Suriname, Uruguay and Venezuela. The Convention defines the human rights that the ratifying states have agreed to respect and guarantee. The Convention also created the Inter-American Court of Human Rights and established the functions and procedures of the Court and of the Commission. In addition to examining complaints of violations of the American Convention against countries who are parties to the Convention, the IACHR has competence, in accordance with the OAS Charter and with the Commission's Statute, to consider alleged violations of the American Declaration by OAS member states that are not yet parties to the American Convention (IACHR 2011); thus, although the United States is not a party to the Convention, the Commission can hear cases brought by American citizens.

The American Convention on Human Rights lists substantive rights within two chapters. The twenty-three articles of chapter II cover individual civil and political rights due to all persons, including the rights to life (article 4), controversially, this is expanded as 'in general, from the moment of conception'; to humane treatment; to a fair trial; to privacy; to freedom of conscience; freedom of assembly; freedom of movement, etc. Chapter III contains a single article covering economic, social and cultural rights; this limited treatment was expanded some ten years later with the Protocol of San Salvador which covers such areas as the right to work, the right to health (article 10), the right to a healthy environment (article 11), the right to food and the right to education; thus far this Protocol has been ratified by only fourteen of the twenty-four states who have ratified the full convention.

Any person, group of persons or non-governmental entity that is legally recognised in one or more OAS member states may petition the Commission with regard to the violation of any right protected by the American Convention, by the American Declaration or by any other pertinent instrument. Also, under the terms of Article 45 of the American Convention, the IACHR may consider communications from a state alleging rights violations by another state. Petitions may be filed in any of the four official languages of the OAS (English, French, Spanish or Portuguese) by the alleged victim of the rights violation or by a third party or, in the case of interstate petitions, by a government.

The IACHR publishes reports documenting its activities comprehensively on its website, these include country reports, topic-based reports and reports on individual cases. Comprehensive annual reports are also produced; these contain a summary of cases and petitions and their follow-up. Reports and the website are available in French, Spanish and Portuguese as well as English.

Petitions to the Commission

There are a number of conditions that those presenting petitions to the Commission must satisfy. First the petitioner must have exhausted all avenues open for remedying the situation in the country concerned, or it must be shown that this has been tried, and failed due to lack of adequate due process, denial of access to remedies or undue delay in decision. Once domestic remedies are exhausted, the petition must be presented within six months of the final decision in the domestic proceedings. If domestic remedies have not been exhausted, the petition must be presented within a reasonable time after the occurrence of the events complained of. The petition must also fulfil other minimal formal requirements which are set out in the Convention and the rules of procedure of the Commission.

When the Commission receives a petition which meets, in principle, all requirements, a number is assigned to the petition and its processing as a case begins. This decision to open a case does not prejudge the Commission's eventual decision on the admissibility or the merits of the case. Once a case is opened, the pertinent parts of the petition are sent to the government with a request for relevant information. During the processing of the case, each party is asked to comment on the responses of the other party. The Commission also may undertake its own investigations, which may include visits, and requests for specific information from parties involved. The Commission may also hold a hearing during the processing of the case, in which both parties are present. In almost every case, the Commission will also offer to assist the parties in negotiating a friendly settlement if they wish.

When the Commission decides that it has sufficient information, the processing of a case is completed. The Commission then prepares a report which includes its conclusions and also generally provides recommendations to the state concerned. This report is not public. The Commission gives the state a period of time to resolve the situation and to comply with the recommendations of the Commission. Upon the expiration of this period of time granted to the state, the Commission has two options. The Commission may prepare a second report, which is generally similar to the initial report and which also generally contains conclusions and recommendations. In this case, the state is again given a period of time to resolve the situation and to comply with the recommendations of the Commission, if such recommendations are made. At the end of this second period granted to the state, the Commission will usually publish its report, although the Convention does allow the Commission to decide otherwise.

Rather than preparing a second report for publication, the Commission may decide to take the case to the Inter-American Court. This must be done within three months of the date of transmission of the initial report to the state concerned. The initial report of the Commission will be attached to the application to the Court. The Commission will appear in all proceedings before the Court. The decision as to whether a case should be submitted to the Court or published is made according to the Commission's judgement about what is in the best interests of human rights.

The recommendations made by the Commission can be very wide-ranging, including directions for the provision of services, resources and compensation to individuals affected, as well as recommendations regarding the policy and laws of the country against which the case is found. Recommendations are binding on member states, but enforcement lies with the state itself. Monitoring therefore is an important part of efforts to ensure full compliance with recommendations. The Commission follows up in detail the response of the member state to recommendations, publishing details of progress or lack of it in its annual reports and on their website.

The Court

According to its Statute, the Court is an autonomous judicial institution, whose purpose is the interpretation and application of the American Convention on Human Rights; it is based in San Jose, Costa Rica (Inter-American Court on Human Rights 2011). The Court consists of seven judges, elected in an individual capacity by secret ballot, from candidates suggested by the states parties to the Convention. Judges serve for six years and may be re-elected only once; judges whose terms have expired continue to deal with those cases they have begun to hear. Three different functions of the Court can be distinguished: adjudicatory, advisory and the power to adopt provisional measures. In relation to adjudication, the cases before the Court are started by an application presented either by the IACHR or by a state. The Court's judgments are final and not subject to appeal, but if within ninety days of the notification of the judgment, there is disagreement regarding the sense or scope of the judgment, the Court can issue an interpretation of the judgment upon request of any of the parties involved. From 2006 to 2010, the average duration of the proceedings in cases has been 17.4 months, duration being calculated from the date the case is submitted to the Court to the date that the Court hands down judgment on reparations (Inter-American Court of Human Rights 2011). The Court monitors compliance with judgments.

The advisory function involves the Court responding to consultations made by the member states of the OAS, or the bodies of the OAS. This advisory competence strengthens the capacity of the organisation to solve matters that arise from the application of the Convention, since it allows the bodies of the OAS to consult the Court about relevant matters. Finally, the Court may adopt such provisional measures as considered necessary in cases of extreme gravity and urgency and when necessary in order to avoid irreparable damage to people, both in cases being processed before the Court and in matters that have not yet been submitted to it, upon request of the IACHR. The resolutions that form the provisional measures are supervised by the Court.

Activities of the IACHR and the Court with specific relevance to health

To illustrate the scope of the IACHR and the Court in relation to health particularly, this section considers some examples taken from across the range of the functions of the Commission and the Court. There are also two detailed case studies. The first of these examines some of the interactions between the Pan American Health Organization (PAHO) and the IACHR, and demonstrates the considerable extent

Case study: PAHO and IACHR interactions for health 1982–2007

PAHO, as the regional office of the WHO and the Inter-American specialised organisation for health, has a central role to play in promoting and protecting the right of everyone to the enjoyment of the highest attainable standard of health or 'the right to health' and other related human rights. During the early 1980s, PAHO began to study how human rights norms related to the right to health had been incorporated into the national constitutions of its member states, and how the links between the enjoyment of health and other related human rights and freedoms could be reflected in its goals, objectives and technical collaboration with countries.

- 1982: PAHO and other Regional Offices, in collaboration with WHO and the Council for International Organizations of Medical Sciences, formulated the first *International Ethical Guidelines for Biomedical Research Involving Human Subjects*. This referred to human rights instruments as essential tools to be used in the application and interpretation of general principles of ethics.
- 1989: PAHO published *The Right to Health in the Americas*, reporting that 'health protection' as a human right was protected in nineteen of the thirty-five constitutions of the member states.
- 1990: PAHO learnt that serious violations of human rights were occurring systematically in many countries of the Americas in mental health services. PAHO organised a Regional Conference on the Restructuring of Psychiatric Care in Latin America, held in Caracas, Venezuela, in November 1990. This resulted in the Declaration of Caracas, which proposed the restructuring of mental health care in a manner consistent with international human rights instruments. Bolis (2002) identifies that the Caracas Declaration was successful in initiating revision of mental health legislation, as well as contributing to a new framework for advocacy in the defence of the rights of mental health patients, but stresses that the process is not yet complete.
- 2006: following the principles established in the Declaration of Caracas, issuing of *Disability: Prevention and Rehabilitation in the Context of the Right to the Enjoyment of the Highest Attainable Standard of Health and Other Related Rights*, to explain the most important links between health and human rights in accordance with human rights treaties, standards, recommendations, technical guidelines, and decisions of human rights bodies.
- 2007: *Health Agenda for the Americas 2008–17* was issued by the Ministers of Health of the Americas in Panama City, renewing commitment to the right to health.
- 2007: PAHO member states adopted the Declaration of Buenos Aires, *Towards a Health Strategy for Equity, Based on Primary Care*, in which 'they committed to taking the principles of the primary health care strategy into account for structuring their health systems for all persons and achieving

> the enjoyment of the highest attainable standard of health, which is a fundamental basic right of every human being'.
>
> (PAHO's e-learning course on health and human rights at http://new.paho.org/hq/index.php?option=com_content&task=view&id=1774&Itemid=1565 accessed May 2011; IACHR 2001, 2009b, 2011)

to which this joint work has resulted in human rights being kept at the forefront of health policy in the Americas. The second case study looks at the rights of people living with HIV/AIDS and shows the important role of the IACHR in improving access to services, in this case ARV.

The IACHR has been particularly active in women's health, most specifically in tackling gender-based violence, and in reproductive health. Cabal et al. (2003) provide a useful overview of cases brought regarding rape and domestic violence. The cases of rape brought before the Commission have often involved the detention and rape of women by military personnel. Cases concerned with rape by doctors within the health system have resulted in legislative and administrative measures to improve the treatment of rape survivors and the provision of services to them. Cases brought in connection with domestic violence have succeeded in winning compensation for the complaints, but also changes in policy and practice in the countries concerned. Experience from cases regarding reproductive health is also growing, and the importance of this area has led IACHR to produce a publication (IACHR 2010) which sets out the duties of the states in guaranteeing women's human rights without discrimination in terms of access by women to maternal health services. It contains specific recommendations in terms of legislation, public policies and services.

In its latest annual report (IACHR 2011), the IACHR draws attention to a number of issues of concern in the region, which have manifold and multiple effects on health. The first of these is forced displacement of thousands of people, particularly members of indigenous communities, due to the construction of large infrastructure projects and exploitation of natural resources. As they report, in many cases, such projects are carried out without prior consultation with the indigenous peoples affected and without sufficient measures to protect their ancestral lands, in violation of the standards of international law. The IACHR also notes with concern the persistence of structural barriers to indigenous peoples' effective enjoyment of ownership rights over their lands, territories and natural resources, such as the lack of legal recognition of indigenous territories, the appropriation of indigenous lands, the displacement of the original population by non-indigenous owners and the proclamation of protected areas in traditional territories. On this issue, the Inter-American Commission has recently published a report on indigenous and tribal peoples' rights over their ancestral lands and natural resources (IACHR 2009a), which analyses the scope of these rights in the light of the jurisprudence of the inter-American system and puts forward specific guidelines and best practices.

Case study: Rights of people living with HIV/AIDS, IACHR Case 12.249

Jorge was HIV positive, living in El Salvador, head of a non-governmental organisation that works to improve the quality of life and promote the empowerment of those living with HIV/AIDS, their family members and other loved ones. The group strives to protect and defend the human rights of all persons whose lives have been touched by HIV/AIDS.

Jorge and his group filed a petition with the IACHR alleging responsibility on the part of his government for violations of various provisions in binding human rights conventions relating to: the right to life; humane treatment; equal protection before the law; juridical protection; and economic, social and cultural rights (IACHR 2001). This claimed that by not providing Jorge and twenty-six other HIV-positive individuals with the triple therapy medication needed to prevent them from dying and to improve their quality of life, the state has violated the right to life, health and wellbeing of the alleged victims. Following recommendations from the IACHR the state reported to the human rights body the decision to authorise the purchase of medication for the provision of therapy and to adopt measures for strengthening and stepping up activities aimed at preventing the transmission of AIDS through education and the promotion of hygiene and preventive health among sectors most at risk for this disease. Additionally, the government announced its intention to create a fund aimed at purchasing antiretroviral medications for the provision of triple therapy to HIV-infected persons. The national health authorities began administering antiretroviral treatment (IACHR 2009b). According to the last annual report of the IACHR, the case is still being monitored since the legislative changes required by some of the recommendations have not yet been completed.

Regarding the situation of the Afro-descendant population in the hemisphere, the IACHR (2011) confirmed that there are still serious problems of racial discrimination that are reflected in the social exclusion and high rates of poverty that those of African descent continue to endure in many countries of the region. In addition, the IACHR received information regarding other serious violations perpetrated against the Afro-descendant population, ranging from harassment and deprivation of liberty to extrajudicial executions. The IACHR will continue monitoring the situation of the Afro-descendants in the region and in 2011 undertook a series of promotional activities to disseminate their rights as a part of 2011's recognition as the international year of Afro-descendants.

The IACHR (2011) also expressed great concern about systemic discrimination and violence against lesbian, gay, transsexual, bisexual and intersexual (LGTBI) persons in the region, reflecting the persistence of high levels of intolerance in society and the failure of governmental authorities to adopt positive measures to combat that discrimination and violence. It notes that some states still have laws that criminalise the behaviour of LGTBI persons, with criminal penalties ranging from ten years in prison or forced labour to life in prison for consensual sexual behaviour between adults of the same sex. The very existence of laws of this kind perpetuates improper stereotypes, creates fear within the sexually diverse community and fosters impunity for serious crimes committed against that community's members. The Commission calls for the repeal of these laws and for all states in the region to adopt measures to promote the enjoyment of human rights by all persons under conditions of equality and respect for decisions regarding the private life of every human being.

Another priority challenge is to protect the right of children and adolescents to live free of violence and discrimination. During 2010 IACHR (2011) reports receiving information regarding abusive practices in state-controlled institutions such as psychiatric institutions, boarding schools, and displaced persons' camps. For this reason, the Commission is currently preparing, in collaboration with the Office of the High Commissioner for Human Rights and UNICEF, a report on juvenile justice in the Americas and a regional report on the situation of institutionalised children. The Commission also reiterates the need for joint and immediate action by the member states to address the problem of corporal punishment. The solution is to legally, explicitly and absolutely prohibit it in all areas and additionally to adopt preventive, educational and other suitable measures to ensure the eradication of this form of violence.

During 2010 women and girls in the region continued to be the victims of gender-based violence and discrimination (IACHR 2011). The right of women to live free of violence and discrimination has been established as a priority challenge, both at a regional and an international level, and the Commission has noted in reiterated opportunities that real access to judicial guarantees and protection is indispensable for the eradication of the problem of violence against women, and for this reason, for the states to effectively comply with their international obligation to act with due diligence *vis-à-vis* this serious problem. Regarding economic, social and cultural rights, discrimination against women continues to be reflected in the labour market; their limited access to social security; their high illiteracy rates compared to men; in the serious poverty, social exclusion and in particular in the limited political participation faced by indigenous and Afro-descendant women. In this respect, the Commission emphasised the need to give priority to caring for women who suffer the consequences of armed conflict or are subject to multiple forms of discrimination and subordination due to race, ethnic origin or poverty. Further, in relation to the right to health of women, the Commission calls upon member states to adopt measures to guarantee this right in order to reduce the high rates of maternal mortality currently existing in the Americas, the principal causes of which are preventable. The right to personal integrity is closely tied to the right to health, given that the provision of adequate and timely maternal health services is one of the principal measures for guaranteeing women's right to personal integrity.

Finally, in direct relation to health, the IACHR (2011) expresses its concern for the serious conditions in which the persons deprived of liberty find themselves, in facilities that are insufficient and inadequate: with serious overcrowding; with no access to drinkable water; with food inadequate in quantity and quality; with no access to health and sanitary services, education and rehabilitation services. The Commission call for states to design public policies directed at guaranteeing the effective enjoyment of the rights of persons deprived of liberty in conformity with the standards identified in the *Principles and Best Practices on the Protection of Persons Deprived of Liberty in the Americas*, which was adopted by the Commission in Resolution 01/08.

Asia-Pacific

The Association of Southeast Asian Nations (ASEAN) was established in 1967; the current ten member states are Brunei Darussalam, Cambodia, Indonesia, Lao PDR, Malaysia, Myanmar, Philippines, Singapore, Thailand and Vietnam. In terms of international human rights treaties, to this point only two conventions have been ratified by all of ASEAN member states, the Convention on the Rights of the Child and the Convention on the Elimination of All Forms of Discrimination Against Women. Four of the ten ASEAN countries have entered reservations to these conventions, which have significantly impacted their applicability within the states concerned.

The ASEAN Intergovernmental Commission on Human Rights (AICHR) was set up in 2009 based on article 14 of the ASEAN Charter, with a remit for promoting and protecting human rights. Item 4 of the AICHR's terms of reference (ASEAN 2009), covering mandate and functions, charges the AICHR with developing an ASEAN Human Rights Declaration, as well as with other functions covering public education on human rights, research, studies and other functions connected with promoting and protecting human rights. A history of its creation can be found in Yen (2011). NGOs in the region recognise that AICHR has only been in existence for a short time and welcome elements in the work plan, such as a programme of thematic studies and the work towards an Asian Charter (SAPA TFAHR 2010), however they point to areas of concern, namely lack of openness and transparency, lack of dedicated secretariat of sufficient size, lack of adequate budget, lack of adequate consultation and failure to adopt rules of procedure. The last is particularly important as this means the Commission cannot officially receive cases alleging human rights violations as the procedures by which they will be addressed have not been agreed. Kelsall (2009), in her analysis of the Commission, points out that the terms of reference adopted in July 2009 limits the Commission's role to that of an advisory body for the ASEAN Secretariat and member states, rather than giving the commission independent enforcement powers. She points out though that work towards an Asian Charter of Human Rights provides a good opportunity for creation of a framework for human rights promotion and protection that is agreed amongst the member states, if it is taken to the point of a legally binding convention. Meijknecht and DeVries (2010) identify a further limitation of the Charter and terms of reference in their lack of any explicit mention of minorities or indigenous peoples, despite recognition of cultural diversity, and their analysis of the reservations made by ASEAN members states to the Convention on the Rights of the Child suggests these are detrimental to children of minorities and indigenous peoples; Meijknecht and De Vries link this to the collectivist and assimilationist character of the 'Asian values' underlying the operation of ASEAN. Finally, Ginbar's (2010) analysis finds the terms of reference unbalanced in terms of an emphasis on promotion, understood in fairly restricted terms of awareness-raising and promoting ratification of international human rights instruments, and not on protection of human rights. Ginbar's analysis concludes by expressing caution about the nature of the ASEAN Declaration on Human Rights that may emerge, fearing that it will be so riddled with 'restrictions, caveats and provisos' as to be worse than not having a regional instrument; Ginbar expresses the hope that the national and regional civil society organisations that have been active in the region so far will prevent this from happening.

There is a wide range of regional NGOs addressing human rights issues in the region. One particularly important body is Forum-Asia, the Asian Forum for Human Rights and Development. This is a regional human rights organisation with forty-seven member organisations across Asia, in seventeen countries: Bangladesh, Cambodia, India, Indonesia, Japan, Malaysia, Mongolia, Myanmar, Nepal, Pakistan, Philippines, Singapore, South Korea, Sri Lanka, Taiwan, Timor-Leste, Thailand. Forum-Asia is a membership-based regional human rights organisation committed to the promotion and protection of all human rights including the right to development. Forum-Asia was founded in 1991 in Manila and its regional Secretariat has been located in Bangkok since 1994. Membership is open to independent, non-profitable, non-partisan, non-violent and non-governmental civil society organisations working in the field of human rights and human development in Asia. The organisation must have been in existence for at least two years. Forum-Asia is the co-convenor of Solidarity for Asian People's Advocacy Task Force on ASEAN and Human Rights (SAPA TFAHR). Forum-Asia and SAPA TFAHR have been active in terms of raising thematic issues and specific cases of human rights violations to the AICHR; these include a submission on the removal of mandatory HIV testing for migrant workers presented to the AICHR meeting in September 2010, and submissions on the rights of women, migrant workers and press freedom. These are fully documented in SAPA TFAHR (2010).

Europe

Within Europe there are two separate (though interlinked) systems to consider, one associated with the Council of Europe and the other with the EU. The Council of Europe's European Convention on Human Rights (ECHR) was signed in 1950 and entered into force in 1953; its original title was the Convention for the Protection of Human Rights and Fundamental Freedoms. The European Court of Human Rights, set up in 1959, covers forty-seven Council of Europe member states that have ratified the convention; a detailed history can be found in Goldhaber (2007).

Individuals or states can apply to the Court alleging violation of the ECHR, and judgments made by the Court are binding on countries concerned. National laws in Europe have been overturned on the grounds that they contravene the European Convention on Human Rights (Neuwahl and Rosas 1995). The Court's jurisdiction in relation to health is limited, since the Convention on Human Rights does not contain a specific article on the right to health or the right to health care. An analysis of the cases dealt with by the court over the period 1959 to 2010 (European Court of Human Rights 2011) is summarised in Table 3.2; as this shows, the articles most often involved are those relating to timely access to justice (right to a fair trial, length of proceedings), followed by protection of property and right to liberty and security.

In relation to health the examples given in the country fact sheets published online do illustrate the potential of cases brought in terms of supporting access to health care for groups like prisoners (alleging violations of article 2 on right to life and article 3 on right to freedom from torture and inhuman or degrading treatment

Table 3.2 Outcome of judgements and types of violation found by European Court of Human Rights, 1959–2010

Total number of judgements	13697★
Percentage of judgments finding at least one violation	83%
Percentage of judgments finding no violation	6%
Percentage of friendly settlements/striking out judgments	8%
Percentage of other judgments (just satisfaction, revision judgments, preliminary objections and lack of jurisdiction)	3%
Percentage of judgments with violation in respect of:	
Length of proceedings	33%
Right to a fair trial	25%
Protection of property	18%
Right to liberty and security	14%
Right to an effective remedy	10%
Inhuman or degrading treatment	6%
Right to respect for private and family life	5%
Freedom of expression	3%
Lack of effective investigation	3%
Right to life – deprivation of life	2%
Lack of effective investigation	2%
Prohibition of discrimination	1%
Freedom of assembly and association	1%
Non enforcement	1%
Prohibition of torture	1%
Other articles of the Convention	2%

★ includes 13 judgements involving 2 states

or punishment) and action against pollution (alleging violation of the right to life, article 2). The EU Network of Independent Experts on Fundamental Rights (EU Network 2006) contrasts the strong approach of the UN Human Rights Committee to the right to life, including the obligation to take all possible measures to reduce infant mortality, to increase life expectancy, to eliminate malnutrition and epidemics, and to prohibit nuclear weapons, to the more cautious approach by the European Court of Human Rights. They note however that, in recent years, the Court has accepted some obligations in relation to serious environmental and health risks. In respect of persons for whom the state has a particular responsibility, such as detainees, persons with disabilities, the elderly or children, in support of the positive obligation to protect the right to life and to prevent certain risks, the European Court of Human Rights has, for instance, found violations of article 2 (the right to life) of the ECHR in cases where detainees were not effectively protected against violence by other inmates or did not enjoy sufficient medical support in case of suicidal tendencies. While states are bound to uphold the rights in the ECHR, as Keller and Sweet (2008) argue, the Court has no authority to invalidate legal norms and its capacity to control change within states is weak at best.

In recent years, the Court's caseload, relative to its capacity to deliver judgments has become unsustainable (FRA 2010b), causing delays in the resolution of cases. Court statistics show a tremendous number of pending applications, 152,000 in total as at 30 April 2011, with ten states (Russia, Turkey, Italy, Ukraine, Poland, Romania, Serbia, Bulgaria, Moldova and Slovenia) accounting for 78 per cent of these (although only 49 per cent of the population), and the remaining 22 per cent lying with the other thirty-seven states.

Turning to the EU, the Charter of Fundamental Rights of the European Union (EU 2000) was proclaimed in Nice in December 2000 (Peers and Ward 2004). Initially its powers amount to 'soft' law, rules of conduct that have no legally binding force (Trubek and Trubek 2005). The Charter contains some fifty-four articles divided into seven titles. The first six titles deal with substantive rights (under the headings of dignity, freedoms, equality, solidarity, citizens' rights and justice), while the last title deals with the interpretation and application of the Charter. Much of the Charter is based on the ECHR, the case-law of the European Court of Justice and pre-existing provisions of European Union law.

Since coming into force in 2009, the Treaty of Lisbon (December 2007) has changed the status of the EU Charter of Fundamental Rights, so that the charter provisions now become 'general principles' of EU law and this means that both EU and member states, when implementing EU law, will need to comply with the EU Charter (FRA 2010a). Several EU states insisted upon a protocol governing national application of the charter in their case, including the UK, Poland and the Czech Republic, although interpretations differ as to exactly what this protocol will actually mean in practice. While Jirasek (2008) argues that the protocol will act as an opt-out that excludes the application of the Charter to Poland and the United Kingdom, Pernice (2008) argues that the protocol is an interpretative protocol which will either have limited or no legal consequences. The explanation offered on the website of the European Commission in its Justice section (accessed 6 May 2011) is that the Union institutions (e.g. the European Commission, the Council and the European Parliament) must respect the rights enshrined in the Charter. The Charter also applies to member states but only when they implement Union law. The Charter's provisions do not extend the EU's competences as defined in the Treaties. The European Union cannot intervene in fundamental rights issues in areas over which, according to the Treaty, it has no competence. The Lisbon Treaty also provides for the legal basis for the European Union to accede to the European Convention on Human Rights which will make the European Court of Human Rights in Strasbourg competent to review acts of the EU institutions. The same website emphasises that the European Commission has no general powers to intervene in individual cases of alleged violations of fundamental rights. It can intervene only when EU law comes into play (for example, when EU legislation is adopted or when a national measure applies an EU law in a manner incompatible with the Charter). McHale (2010) in her analysis identifies that, although the Charter potentially has considerable implications for health law and health policy throughout the EU, it is uncertain whether the EU Charter will make any considerable difference over the long term. The Charter contains, in article 35, the right to health care, stated as: 'Everyone has the right of access to preventive health care and the right to benefit from medical treatment under the conditions established by national laws and practices. A high level of human health protection shall be ensured in the definition and implementation of all Union policies and activities.'

The European Union Agency for Fundamental Rights (FRA) is an advisory body of the European Union. It was established in 2007 by a legal act of the European Union and is based in Vienna, Austria, and replaced an earlier organisation, the European Monitoring Centre for Racism and Xenophobia (McHale 2010). The FRA helps to ensure that fundamental rights of people living in the EU are protected. It does this by collecting evidence about the situation of fundamental rights across the European Union and providing advice, based on evidence, about how to improve the situation. The FRA also informs people about their fundamental rights. In doing so, it helps to make fundamental rights a reality for everyone in the European Union. As McHale (2010) points out, however, its role does not extend to systematic permanent monitoring of human rights in member states. The annual reports of the FRA do provide an insight into the situation in the European Union, although, drawing as they do on the specific projects they have recently completed, the overview they offer is by no means a comprehensive analysis. Their most recent annual report (FRA2010a) highlights the problems of discrimination against ethnic and sexual minorities; in the case of ethnic minorities this discrimination is manifest in reduced access to housing, education, employment and health care. The report also identifies that many equality bodies and national human rights institutions lack resources, independence and often have very weak mandates. It remains to be seen how influential the FRA will prove in encouraging EU member states to address the problems identified.

Middle East

The Middle East is another region with a system that has been much less developed since the 1940s; reasons for this can be located in its frequently turbulent political history. A Permanent Arab Commission on Human Rights (PACHR) was founded in September 1968 by the Council of the League of Arab States (Encyclopaedia Britannica 2011). The work of the PACHR has been preoccupied primarily with the rights of Arabs living in Israeli-occupied territories. The Arab Charter on human rights was adopted by the Council of the League of Arab States in September 1994, but never came into force. The Charter contains a specific article in relation to culture and religion for minorities, stating: 'Minorities shall not be deprived of their right to enjoy their culture or to follow the teachings of their religions.'

The Charter includes no specific mention of health or the right to health but articles 38 and 39 deal with health matters for the family, and young persons respectively, stating:

Article 38
(a) The family is the basic unit of society, whose protection it shall enjoy.
(b) The State undertakes to provide outstanding care and special protection for the family, mothers, children and the aged.

Article 39
Young persons have the right to be afforded the most ample opportunities for physical and mental development.

The Charter was the subject of considerable criticism by NGOs and IGOs (Mann 2004). These criticisms pointed out that it does not correspond to many international human rights standards as set forth in previous international declarations and treaties, particularly the Universal Declaration of Human Rights. A process of modernising the Charter then took place, and although this has addressed some of the concerns, some remain, including the possibility of sentencing people under 18 years of age to death, allowing for non-discrimination laws that are applicable only for citizens, and limitations on the freedom of expression and association and gender equality (Mann 2004). During the Arab Summit held in Tunis in May 2004, a 'modernised' version of the Arab Charter on Human Rights was adopted. The revised document represents a major improvement over the Charter of 1994, affirming the principles contained in the UN Charter, the International Bill of Rights and the Cairo Declaration on Human Rights in Islam (discussed in the next section). The Charter, which entered into force in March 2008 (Rishmawi 2010), contains a number of traditional human rights as well as provisions of a more political nature. As Rishmawi (2010) identifies, the real test of the Arab Human Rights Committee set up to fulfil monitoring functions will come when it considers the first reports from countries; no further updated report in English was available as at May 2011.

In a report on the state of human rights in the Arab Region in 2008, the Cairo Institute for Human Rights Studies (CIHRS 2008) reported that the status of human rights there had increasingly worsened. Their latest report, released in March 2011 (CIHRS 2010), identifies a further worsening in the situation, and also argues that the League of Arab States is working to undermine the UN human rights system and standards. CIHRS (2010) is similarly critical of the OIC (Organisation of the Islamic Cooperation), which is considered next.

Organisation of Islamic Cooperation

The Organisation of Islamic Cooperation (OIC), formerly the Organisation of the Islamic Conference, is the second largest intergovernmental organisation after the United Nations. It currently has a membership of fifty-seven states from four continents. The Organisation aims to be the collective voice of the Muslim world and to safeguard and protect the interests of the Muslim world in the spirit of promoting international peace and harmony among various peoples of the world. The Organisation was established in a summit meeting which took place in Morocco in September 1969 following the arson attack on Al-Aqsa Mosque in Jerusalem. The present Charter of the Organisation was adopted by the Eleventh Islamic Summit held in Dakar in March 2008. The Organisation has consultative and cooperative relations with the UN and other intergovernmental organisations to protect the vital interests of the Muslims, and to work for the settlement of conflicts and disputes involving member states. In 2005, the OIC adopted a Ten-Year Program of Action which envisages joint action by member states, promotion of tolerance and moderation, modernisation, extensive reforms in all spheres of activities including science and technology, education, trade enhancement, and emphasises good governance and promotion of human rights in the Muslim world, especially with regard to rights of children, women and elderly and the family values enshrined by Islam.

Under the Charter, the Organisation's aims include: reaffirming support for the rights of peoples as stipulated in the UN Charter and international law: member states shall uphold and promote, at the national and international levels, good governance, democracy, human rights and fundamental freedoms, and the rule of law. The OIC adopted the Cairo Declaration on Human Rights in Islam in 1990, and the Covenant on the Rights of the Child in Islam in 2004; however there are as yet no reporting or monitoring mechanisms to examine implementation in member states. There has been some discussion about setting up a Permanent Commission on Human Rights within the OIC (Shaikh 2009) but this has not happened yet.

Regional systems: developments into the future

As is clear from the sections above, regional systems in relation to human rights are nowhere fully developed and, arguably, it is far too early to show how effective their operations may prove to be in protecting and promoting human rights. Like the global system, considerable time delays can be seen between the lodging of complaints and the rulings and decisions of the relevant bodies. A further challenge is the volume of cases accumulating in the systems. The system in Americas perhaps shows the most positive effects in terms of promoting change in member countries, and it is perhaps no coincidence that this system is the one with the most thorough system of monitoring implementation of recommendations. It is also notable that much has been achieved through the joint work with the regional office of the World Health Organization for the Americas, PAHO.

4 National and subnational human rights systems

This chapter turns to the question of national and subnational systems for protection and promotion of human rights. There is incredible diversity here, and the chapter cannot attempt to cover every country and its system in detail. Instead, it discusses five different countries to illustrate some of the different approaches and structures that are found, and in each case to explore links to health and health policy.

Nowadays, usually a national system is based around some kind of national human rights institution (NHRI), in some cases there is more than one institution. As Pohjolainen's fascinating exploration of the history of these bodies demonstrates (2006), the present concept and status of NHRIs developed over a period of fifty years, and is closely linked to the growth and development of international human rights, in particular based around the UN system. Historically, Pohjolainen divides this evolution into three broad stages: the introduction and development of the idea (1946–78), the 'popularisation' of the concept (1978–90), and the expansion of national human rights institutions (from 1990 onwards). She notes that the end of the cold war and the collapse of Communism were significant factors in the developmental process. Pohjolainen's analysis demonstrates that it was only in the early 1990s that governments came to accept the principle that all national institutions should fulfil certain minimum criteria. A crucial step in this process came in 1993 when the World Conference on Human Rights endorsed the establishment of national institutions (UN General Assembly 1993) and the use of the 'Principles relating to the status of national institutions' that had been formulated in 1991 and are generally known as the Paris Principles after the city where they were formulated, see Table 4.1 for a summary of the principles. Pohjolainen (2006) demonstrates that the UN has played an important role in the development and establishment of national human rights structures by functioning both as an intergovernmental arena and as a human rights actor; while the UN has not worked in a vacuum, she considers its role has been decisive. A collection of papers edited by Lindsnaes *et al.* (2000), and published by the NHRI for Denmark, the Danish Centre for Human Rights, offers an interesting analysis of the early years of experience gained in developing institutions in line with the Paris Principles and illustrates some of the challenges institutions face in ensuring independence, sufficient budget and public awareness of their existence.

Table 4.1 Main features of the Paris principles for NHRIs

1.	Has a broadly defined mandate with emphasis on the national implementation of international human rights standards
2.	Is established by legislative means
3.	Is independent of the state in decision-making procedures
4.	Has a pluralist representation of civil society and vulnerable groups in its governing body/bodies
5.	Handles complaints from individuals

Source: derived from Chapter 1 of Lindsnaes *et al.* 2000

In the early 1990s there were only relatively few NHRIs (Pohjolainen 2006); this number has risen steadily ever since so that at the time of writing (June 2011) there are 125 NHRIs listed on the database of the National Human Rights Institutions Forum (http://nhri.ohchr.org). Following Pohjolainen (2006) four broad categories can be distinguished in terms of the different models for national human rights institutions: the human rights commission model, the advisory committee model, the ombudsman model and the human rights institute model. She also distinguishes four different functions that NHRIs may have: *monitoring* of observance of human rights, including sometimes the investigation of complaints; *advisory*, providing advice to the government and sometimes to other relevant actors; *education and information*, including awareness-raising, education and training; and finally, *research*, undertaking specific investigations, studies and sometimes public inquiries.

At the national level, possibilities depend on the position of human rights within the country concerned. In some countries the right to health or similar rights have been established in national constitutions, others have utilised non-binding policies instead, limiting recourse to national courts. A recent survey by the OHCHR (2009a) of the National Human Rights Institutions (NHRIs) linked into the OHCHR's network of NHRIs finds that a large majority of NHRIs are under twenty years old. Each of the four regions distinguished by the OHCHR showed a different type of institution dominating: mainly statute-based commissions in Asia-Pacific and Europe, with the ombudsman model being common in Eastern Europe; mainly constitutionally based commissions in Africa; and mainly constitutionally based ombuds-institutions in the Americas (OHCHR 2009a).

The next section presents five different national human rights systems and, following that, the chapter moves on to look at the question of linking NHRIs into the UN system, including a brief discussion of the role of the ICC, the International Coordinating Committee of NHRIs. The chapter concludes with an examination of the success of national human rights systems in terms of the promotion and protection of human rights.

Contrasts and convergences

Within this section, five countries are considered: Sweden, Ghana, Australia, India and Japan. The countries discussed have been chosen to illustrate some of the different mandates, structures and implementation mechanisms in existence. In each case the latest annual report of the relevant national agency, if available, has been used to give an illustration of the scope and activities of the agency.

Sweden: the precursor of modern NHRIs

Carver (2010) identifies the Swedish system, based on the Swedish Ombudsman, as the precursor of all modern NHRIs. The Swedish Ombudsman was set up in 1809, when the Swedish Parliament created a new official known as the Justitie-Ombudsman. This loosely translates as 'citizen's defender' or 'representative of the people'; the responsibilities of the Justitie-Ombudsman were to ensure that public authorities and their staff comply with the laws and other statutes governing their actions. This supervision was exercised by evaluating and investigating complaints from the general public, by making inspections of the various authorities and by conducting other forms of inquiry that they initiate themselves. In Swedish the word 'ombudsman' is without gender and can indicate a person of either sex.

Before 1 May 2009, the Swedish national human rights system was based around four different Ombudsmen: the Children's Ombudsman, the Swedish Ombudsman against Ethnic Discrimination, the Swedish Disability Ombudsman and finally the Ombudsman for Equal Rights. On 1 May 2009, a single agency was created, the Equality Ombudsman (DO). This is a government agency that seeks to combat discrimination and promote equal rights and opportunities for everyone. In pursuit of this goal, the agency is primarily concerned with ensuring compliance with the Discrimination Act (Equality Ombudsman 2011). This law prohibits discrimination related to a person's sex, transgender identity or expression, ethnicity, religion or other belief, disability, sexual orientation or age. The government appoints the head of the agency.

The Ombudsman's principal task is to ensure compliance with the Discrimination Act. The Ombudsman registers and investigates complaints based on the law's prohibition of discrimination and harassment, and can represent victims in court free of charge. The Ombudsman also investigates complaints from employees on parental leave who feel they have been treated unfairly for having taken such leave. In addition, the Ombudsman exercises supervision by monitoring how employers, higher education institutions and schools live up to the provisions of the Discrimination Act requiring active measures against discrimination. The Ombudsman's other duties include raising awareness and disseminating knowledge and information about discrimination and about the prohibitions against discrimination, both among those who risk discriminating against others and those who risk being subjected to discrimination. This means that the agency offers guidance to employers, higher education institutions, schools and others, and helps develop useful methods on their behalf. A further task is to ensure, through awareness-raising initiatives, that everyone knows their rights. In addition, the Ombudsman is required to draw attention and create debate around human rights issues. The DO also has special responsibility for reporting on new research and international developments in the human rights and discrimination field.

One particular issue addressed has been the issue of national minorities, and in particular, the Sami people, this is an issue that was raised in the context of the Universal Periodic Review of Sweden at the UN (HRCl 2010). The Sami were recognised by Sweden as an indigenous people in 1977, and as such should enjoy certain additional rights under Swedish national law as well as international law (Pikkarainen and Brodin 2008a). Research commissioned by the Ombudsman against Ethnic Discrimination (reported in Pikkarainen and Brodin 2008a) revealed that the Sami continue to experience discrimination in all areas of society, including in access to health and health services, and that institutionalised racism or structural discrimination exists widely. Recommendations proposed by the Equality Ombudsman were directed to the Swedish government and include the ratification of relevant conventions on indigenous peoples; a future programme of work for the agency in this area was also set up. A second report (Pikkarainen and Brodin 2008b) examined discrimination against national minorities in the education system, and put forward a wide-ranging set of recommendations to address the issue, both inside and outside the education system.

Sweden was the first country in the world to introduce a legal ban on discrimination associated with gender identity or gender expression; this took effect in January 2009 (Equality Ombudsman 2010). Previous anti-discrimination legislation only protected the right of transsexuals not to be subjected to discrimination. The new ground of discrimination was introduced to ensure comprehensive protection against discrimination for all transpersons, including transvestites, intersexuals and intergender and transgender persons.

Ghana: linking human rights and anti-corruption

The Commission on Human Rights and Administrative Justice (CHRAJ) is an independent organisation for the safeguarding of human rights in Ghana. It was established in 1993 by an act of the Parliament of Ghana (Commission of Human Rights Act, 1993 (Act 456) [Ghana], 6 July 1993, available at www.unhcr.org/refworld/docid/44bf7f804.html, accessed May 2011) as directed by Article 216 of the 1992 Ghana constitution. The CHRAJ is a constitutional body and can formulate its own rules of procedure (Quashigah 2000).

Since its inception, cases handled by CHRAJ range from human rights abuses and corruption to administrative injustice (Asibuo 2001). Asibuo's scrutiny of the Commission's performance over the period 1993 to 1999 leads him to conclude that it has been successful in terms of keeping the executive arm of government on its toes in terms of both human rights and public accountability. He also notes that CHRAJ has been ambitious both in creating a nationwide network of offices and in taking on a broad array of issues, though the heavy workload and the poor conditions of service have led to high staff turnover.

In its independent submission to Ghana's UPR under the UN system (CHRAJ 2008), the Commission notes that, although there has been a distinct improvement in the promotion and protection of human rights in Ghana and that there has been a positive increase in space for discourse regarding human rights and much greater tolerance for freedom of expression, there are still particular problems with respect to achievement of access to health care, domestic violence and the rights of women and children. According to the *Accra Daily Mail* (8 September 2010) Mr Emile Short, the Commissioner for Human Rights and Administrative Justice at the time, proposed the separation of the mandates of the commission, as they are 'overly broad'. His views run counter to other commentators such as Kumar (2006) who argues that corruption is a major issue in developing countries and should be perceived as a human rights issue where it acts as a serious impediment to governance. Recent information on the work of CHRAJ is hard to find, their website remained unavailable throughout the period May to October 2011, and their annual reports could not be located.

Australia: 'Human rights: everyone, everywhere, everyday'

Australia provides an interesting example of a country that has regional differences within the country in relation to human rights. Australia is a federal system with some variation between states; one of the complexities of life in Australia is disentangling commonwealth from state responsibilities in areas including health and human services provision. The Australian constitution does not guarantee human rights; successive Australian governments have argued in the various periodic reports submitted to the UN system that separate legislation covers these adequately. A Human Rights and Equal Opportunity Commission was established in 1986 by an act of the federal Parliament. The Commission is an independent statutory organisation and reports to the federal Parliament through the Attorney-General. Over the period 2008–9 the Human Rights and Equal Opportunity Commission changed its name to the Australian Human Rights Commission, with the vision of 'Human rights: everyone, everywhere, everyday'.

Complaints can be brought in relation to 'discrimination, harassment or bullying' and in relation to breach of human rights by the Commonwealth and its agencies according to the Commission's website (www.humanrights.gov.au/complaints_information/index.html, accessed May 2011). Note that this does not contain any provision for complaints to be brought under the national system in relation to human rights breaches (apart from discrimination) by private companies or other levels of government or individuals, as the Commission explicitly points out in its annual report (AHRC 2010a: 61), thus falling somewhat short of the scope implied by the Commission's vision. The Commission offers a conciliation process for complaints. If the complaint is not resolved by conciliation, and the President of the Commission is satisfied that a complaint cannot be resolved, the complaint will be terminated. In some cases, the complainant can then make an application within the next sixty days for the Federal Magistrates Court or the Federal Court of Australia for the court to hear the allegations in the complaint. Complaints lodged under the Australian Human Rights Commission Act, which allege a breach of human rights or discrimination in employment by or on behalf of the Commonwealth, cannot be taken to court for determination. If conciliation is unsuccessful or inappropriate, and the Commission finds that there has been a breach of human rights or workplace discrimination has occurred, then the Commission can prepare a report of the complaint, including recommendations for action, for the Attorney General. The reports must be tabled in Parliament, and are available on the Commission's website.

In the year 2009–10, the Commission received 2,517 complaints and finalised 2,426, 50 per cent were successfully conciliated, 18 per cent were withdrawn or discontinued and the remaining 32 per cent were terminated or declined with no further details of outcome given (AHRC 2010a). In 2009–10, 42 per cent of complaints received were lodged under the Disability Discrimination Act, 22 per cent under the Racial Discrimination Act, 21 per cent under the Sex Discrimination Act, 8 per cent under the Australian Human Rights Commission Act and 7 per cent under the Age Discrimination Act. The majority of complaints received in 2009–10 under the Australian Human Rights Commission Act related to alleged breaches of the International Covenant on Civil and Political Rights and discrimination in employment on the ground of criminal record; these have been the main subject areas of complaint for the past five years (AHRC 2010a).

The Commission reports a wide range of other activities for the year 2009–10, including the launch of a range of interactive education materials for teachers and secondary students on human rights and completion of two important pieces of work in relation to gender equality (AHRC 2010c) and African Australians (AHRC 2010b). The Commission recommended the establishment of a Human Rights Act during the national consultation held in 2009, but this was not taken up by the government.

Some Australian states, including Victoria, have introduced state-specific initiatives. The main human rights body at state level in Victoria is the Victorian Equal Opportunity and Human Rights Commission (VEOHRC), an independent statutory body with responsibilities under three laws: the Equal Opportunity Act (1995 and 2011), the Racial and Religious Tolerance Act 2001 and the Charter of Human Rights and Responsibilities Act 2006. The Equal Opportunity Acts (1995 and 2011) mean it is against the law to discriminate against people on the basis of a number of different personal characteristics. The Racial and Religious Tolerance Act 2001 makes it against the law to vilify people because of their race or religion. Under the Equal Opportunity Acts (1995 and 2011) and the Racial and Religious Tolerance Act 2001, the Commission helps people resolve complaints of discrimination, sexual harassment and racial or religious vilification through a free and impartial complaint resolution service, with the aim of achieving a mutual agreement.

The Victorian Charter of Human Rights and Responsibilities (Department of Justice 2006) includes twenty specific rights, see Table 4.2. A comparison of Table 4.2 in relation to the UDHR, ICCPR and ICESCR shows that the Victorian Charter is much more limited, for example rights to education, health and employment are not covered. The Charter means that government and public bodies must consider human rights when making laws and providing services. The Commission's role is to educate people about the rights and responsibilities contained in the Charter and to report annually to the government about the operation of the Charter. The Commission does not handle complaints related to the Charter. Complaints about

Table 4.2 Twenty Rights in the Victorian Charter of Rights and Responsibilities

Freedom	Dignity
Freedom from forced work (section 11)	Protection from torture and cruel, inhuman or degrading treatment (section 10)
Freedom of movement (section 12)	Privacy and reputation (section 13)
Freedom of thought, conscience, religion and belief (section 14)	Appropriate treatment of children in the criminal process (section 23)
Freedom of expression (section 15)	Right to a fair hearing (section 24)
Peaceful assembly and freedom of association (section 16)	Rights in criminal proceedings (section 25)
Property rights (section 20)	Right not to be tried or punished more than once (section 26)
Right to liberty and security of person (section 21)	Right not to be prosecuted or punished for things that were not criminal offences at the time they were committed (section 27)
Humane treatment when deprived of liberty (section 22)	
Respect	*Equality*
Right to life (section 9)	Recognition and equality before the law (section 8)
Protection of families and children (section 17)	Taking part in public life (section 18)
Cultural rights (section 19)	

Source: summarised from Department of Justice (2006)

breaches of the Charter can be made to the Victorian Ombudsman if the complaint involves government departments, statutory authorities, local councils or a private agency that carries out statutory responsibilities of government. If the complaint is not covered by the ombudsman, the website directs the reader to a list which, as at 16 May 2011, contains fourteen other Victorian complaint and dispute resolution bodies, four federal complaint and dispute resolution bodies, two specialist police bodies, four Victorian courts and tribunals and eight Commonwealth and interstate ombudsman offices. This certainly does not represent a simple or straightforward system.

In relation to human rights, the VEOHRC reports annually on the operation of the Charter, and carries out a range of advocacy functions, as well as running an advice line and offering training and consultancy. From its latest annual report the Commission delivers a picture of mixed progress, reporting positive change occurring across government agencies, resulting in positive outcomes for Victorians, but identifying that the impact of the Charter across government and local government is inconsistent and that there are instances where, despite policy and legislation complying with human rights obligations, practical implementation and service delivery fail to live up to these (VEOHRC 2011a, 2011b). With particular relevance to health they quote the Department of Health (VEOHRC 2011a: 34) as reporting that the incorporation of human rights considerations in the development of policy relating to restrictive interventions has led to policy that supports reducing restrictive interventions where possible and a proportionate response to prevailing risk. They also report that the Charter resulted in the Public Health and Well Being Act 2008 'being more explicit about the human rights principles underpinning the public health approach' (VEOHRC 2011a: 35).

Under the act establishing the Charter, there are requirements for four- and eight-year reviews of its operation. The four-year review commenced in April 2011, and a report (SARC 2011) was laid before Parliament on 14 September 2011. The scope of the review was broad. It was specifically required to consider whether additional human rights should be included in the Charter, including (but not limited to) economic, social and cultural rights, women's rights and the rights of children, as they are set out in the relevant United Nations Conventions. The review also considered whether to include the right to indigenous self-determination, whether regular auditing of public authorities should be mandatory and whether a direct remedies provision should be added. The VEOHRC has undertaken a range of community consultations on issues relevant to the review, including indigenous self-determination (VEOHRC 2010b), the rights of people with disabilities (VEOHRC 2010c), economic, social and cultural rights (VEOHRC 2010d) and the rights of women (VEOHRC 2010e). The review report finds that the case for adding new categories of rights, reviews and proceedings to the existing Charter has not been made (SARC 2011). The acting Victorian Equal Opportunity and Human Rights Commissioner expressed VEOHRC's disappointment that the majority view in the report recommends a reduction in the obligation on government to take human rights into account in its work, when many of the submissions, from government and the community, including the submissions of the Commission, supported the Charter as a means of enhancing government transparency and accountability (VEOHRC 2011c). The Victorian government has six months to consider its response to the review report.

Australia has ratified all the main UN human rights treaties and Australia's record on human rights is generally regarded as comparatively good, with some important exceptions: indigenous rights; treatment of refugees and asylum seekers and people with disabilities; and provision of mental health services. See for example the documentation for the 2011 Universal Periodic Review for Australia. It also receives criticism for its lack of comprehensive national human rights laws, and lack of attention to the full range of economic and social rights including health care and housing (Lynch 2009; Mapulanga-Hulston and Harpur 2009). The very first policy law of the first federal Parliament was the White Australia Policy and ever since then the Australian government has violated the human rights of Aboriginal people in many ways, including the restriction of movement. Until 1967 Aboriginal people were not allowed access to public places such as pubs, swimming pools and public transport. Aboriginal people experienced widespread discrimination and inequalities. Much of this discrimination was through laws set up to prevent Aboriginal people from participating in society as equals. These laws, practices and attitudes have had economic, social, psychological and political consequences that are still witnessed today. In 2010, the published *Concluding Observations of the Committee on the Elimination of Racial Discrimination on Australia CERD/C/AUS/CO/15–17* noted Australia's acknowledgement that Aboriginal and Torres Straits Islanders occupy a special place in its society as the first peoples of Australia and welcomed the establishment of the National Congress of Australia's First Peoples. However the Committee expressed concern that the National Congress is only an advisory body representing member organisations and individuals and may not be fully representative of Australia's first peoples. They regretted limited progress towards constitutional acknowledgement of Australia's indigenous peoples, and slow implementation of the principle of indigenous peoples' exercising meaningful control over their affairs, and they recommended that the negotiation of a treaty agreement be considered (paragraph 15). The Committee also expressed concern about the Northern Territory Emergency Response (NTER) and its discriminatory impact on affected communities, including restrictions on indigenous rights to land, property, social security, adequate standards of living, cultural development, work and remedies (paragraph 16). A case study on the NTER appears in Chapter 5.

India: the potential of national litigation

Basic human rights are guaranteed in the Indian constitution of 1950, and the Protection of Human Rights Act 1993 in article 2 emphasises that 'human rights means the rights relating to life, liberty, equality and dignity of the individual guaranteed by the Constitution or embodied in the International Covenants and enforceable by courts in India'. The Indian National Human Rights Commission, created in 1993 (Sripati 2000), has quasi-jurisdictional competence, that is, powers to compel the appearance of witnesses and the production of evidence under the Protection of Human Rights Act 1993. The founding statutes of the Indian NHRC explicitly provide that the human rights in their mandate are those derived from international sources, from treaties ratified by the state and incorporated into domestic law. This excludes economic, social and cultural rights, which are not protected in the constitutional Bill of Rights, but have a secondary status as non-enforceable 'directive principles of state policy'. However, according to Kumar (2006) the NHRC has followed the Supreme Court in taking an expansive approach to both the use of treaties as sources of law at the municipal level and in developing the application of economic, social and cultural rights. The Commission itself also reports its role in 'studying treaties and other international instruments on human rights, and making recommendations for their effective implementation' (NHRC 2006: 7). In the latest available commission report, the NHRC reports its view that the right to life with dignity means that 'it is essential for the Commission to focus, in equal measure, on economic, social and cultural rights, just as it does on civil and political rights' (NHRC 2009: 2).

The Human Rights Protection Act, 1993, also provided for State Human Rights Commissions to be created to deal with complaints (NHRC 2006). The NHRC has been pursuing this with the state governments since its inception, however it reports that not all states have functioning commissions (NHRC 2009). Complaints may be brought to the commission by individuals or may be raised by Commissions themselves on the basis of a media report. The Commission can make recommendations and award compensation. One of the functions of the Commission is increasing human rights literacy and promoting knowledge about mechanisms available for rights protection. Two other crucial functions of the Commission linked to its role as a protector are the power to intervene in legal

Case study: Access to palliative care in India

In 2008, Human Rights Watch undertook research into the experiences of those in India requiring palliative care (HRW 2009), including interviewing more than 100 people across India, including patients with advanced life-threatening or debilitating illnesses, health care experts and volunteers, and government health officials. Their research identified that only five out of some 300 medical colleges in the entire country have integrated any instruction into their curricula on palliative care. Consequently, the vast majority of medical doctors in India are unfamiliar with even the most basic tenets of palliative care. In many cases, patients are denied treatment and suffer severe pain, often for weeks or months on end. Many such patients told Human Rights Watch that their suffering was so severe that they wanted to die. Some said they had contemplated or attempted suicide. The report also documented the difference that palliative care made to recipients' quality of life.

The report was published in October 2009. This was followed by activities in partnership with Pallium India and the Pain Relief and Palliative Care Society of Hyderabad, and the creation of detailed proposals for how doctors specialising in palliative care should be trained. These proposals were submitted to the Medical Council of India.

Human Rights Watch also began advising the plaintiffs in a case on palliative care still being heard by India's Supreme Court on how international standards could be used to strengthen their case. This case, brought by the Indian Association of Palliative Care and others, would oblige the government to introduce palliative care training for health care providers and to eliminate drug laws that impede the availability of essential pain medicine.

In January 2011, years of joint advocacy by Human Rights Watch and Indian palliative care groups culminated in the Medical Council of India recognising palliative care as a specialisation of medicine and approving an MD Palliative Care program.

(Compiled from HRW (2009) and www.hrw.org/en/news/2011/02/14/upholding-right-health, accessed May 2011)

proceedings that involve the violation of fundamental rights and the power of initiating new litigation (Sripati 2000).

India provides an excellent example of the potential of the use of national litigation to directly support the right to health. Article 21 of the Indian constitution guarantees an individual's right to life and is enforceable in court. Although the article does not contain any explicit reference to a right to health, in 1981 the Indian Supreme Court signalled its intention to make the right to health enforceable by inference from the right to life. As Sharma (2003) reports, the Supreme Court, following a review of conditions in a number of mental hospitals, gave the Commission the responsibility of monitoring implementation of its recommendations regarding change in three mental hospitals. A sequence of cases (twenty-two separate cases over the period 1980 to 2002 are described in Singh *et al.* 2007) has resulted in courts directing provision of particular services to disadvantaged groups in the population and health-promoting changes in workplaces and working conditions, including:

- installation of safety measures in state-run pencil factories;
- improvements in working conditions in the state- and private-run asbestos industry;
- provision of health services to convicted criminals;
- provision of emergency medical care to all free of charge.

One of the ongoing issues reported in the NHRC's latest report is progress on efforts to improve availability of medical care to the rural populations in India (NHRC 2009).

India is a federal country with twenty-eight states and seven union territories. Average figures for India hide a great deal of variation in the performance of different states in relation to health (Bajpai *et al.* 2010) and in relation to human rights violations (Beer and Mitchell 2006). For an analysis of the various stages in the history of human rights movements in India, see Gudavarthy (2008). Prakasam *et al.* (2010) give an interesting collection of papers presented at the Sixth National Conference of the Indian Association for Social Sciences and Health on the theme 'Health, Equity and Human Rights'; these illustrate that the issue of human rights argumentation in support of public health goals has been taken up very broadly in India, addressing health inequities, maternal health, gender dimensions of health, the reduction of vulnerability, nutrition and health, and finally social aspects of health.

Japan: a system characterised by absence of an NHRI

The 1946 Constitution of Japan (*Nihon Koku Kenpo*) adopted human rights, with a provision on 'fundamental human rights' in article 11. The 1946 Constitution also provides for women's suffrage and the separation of state powers as a principle of democratic Japanese government. As Holland (2009) identifies, the (American) framers of the constitution intended that individual rights would receive protection through the Supreme Court, who have explicit power of judicial review.

Japan has not established a national human rights institution. The Japanese government undertakes human rights promotion and protection work through two major, parallel systems: the Human Rights Bureau under the Ministry of Justice and the Human Rights Volunteers. The Human Rights Bureau works along with eight Human Rights Departments under the Ministry of Justice's Legal Bureaus located in eight major cities in the country. These government human rights bodies deal with 'human rights infringements', which are defined as not only against the law but also against the spirit of respecting human rights, which is the basic principle of the Constitution of Japan and the Universal Declaration of Human Rights. These bodies can undertake 'voluntary' investigation to determine whether or not human rights infringement has occurred based on 'requests' for relief from victims or based on report of newspapers and magazines. Once a human rights infringement has been confirmed, relief measures can be provided, including legal advice, conciliation, strict warning to the perpetrator and assistance to the victim.

Parallel to the existence of the Human Rights Bureau is the group of Human Rights Volunteers (around 14,000 volunteers in total) who are appointed by the Minister of Justice. They are lay people who work to encourage respect for human rights, make efforts to avoid infringements of the rights of residents and to protect human rights in their local community. From among the Human Rights Volunteers, some are appointed as conciliators under the 'Human Rights Conciliator System'. Some are appointed by the Minister of Justice as Volunteers for Children's Rights Protection to deal with problems affecting child rights. The latter collect information on children's rights in addition to promoting cooperation with the PTA (Parents-Teachers Association), Kodomokai (Children's Neighbourhood Associations) and the Commissioner for Children to identify signs of abuse as soon as possible.

The Japanese government (Ministry of Justice n.d.) identifies several human rights issues in the country relating to children (particularly bullying, corporal punishment, child abuse, child prostitution and child pornography), elderly persons, disabled persons, Dowa Issues (or discrimination against the Burakumin), Ainu people (indigenous people in Japan), foreign nationals, HIV carriers, Hansen's disease patients, persons released from prison after serving their sentence, crime victims, people whose human rights are violated using the internet, the homeless, persons with identity disorders and women. The issue of sexual preferences is also listed as a human rights problem. Japanese human rights organisations add other human rights issues involving government officials, such as in the case of *daiyo kangoku* (substitute prison) system and the interrogation process for crime suspects (Joint NGO submission by Japan International Human Rights NGO Network and 51 Signatory Organisations Related to Japan for the Universal Periodic Review, 2nd Session of the United Nations Human Rights Council, scheduled in May 2008: 3).

Japanese human rights organisations (ibid., p. 1) criticise the government for failing to establish an independent national human rights institution. They also cite the inadequacy of the current human rights mechanism in the country. The Human Rights Bureau of the Ministry of Justice, for example, is criticised for most of its personnel working part-time since they hold other positions at the same time. The location of the Human Rights Bureau as part of the Ministry of Justice leads to the argument that this situation provides 'limitations to the remedies available for human rights violations made by the state and bureaucracy', which the Japanese human rights organisations find a 'not uncommon' occurrence (ibid.). According to Japanese government responses in discussions at the UN General Assembly (UN General Assembly 2010), a bill aimed at establishing an independent national human rights institution is under consideration.

Japan thus sits in a very different position in terms of its human rights system than many other countries, and it is therefore of interest to examine the extent to which international systems have an impact within Japan. Iida (2004) presents an analysis of the impact of international human rights law on Japan for three different topics, commercial sexual exploitation of children, eugenics and wartime sexual slavery, and the measures taken to remedy them. The analysis finds that, although international human rights law and norms played a major role in each of these episodes, its influence was uneven. To explain this variation, the analysis focused on the domestic balance of power in Japan and identifies three significant factors: (1) shared common interests between pro-human rights constituencies and their political opponents; (2) consensual decision-making; and (3) transnational coalition-building through international conferences. In terms of the outcomes, Japan was successful in terms of passing a law to tackle commercial sexual exploitation of children, and following this through to prosecution, through an alignment of these three factors. For eugenics, human rights campaigners were targeting Japan's 1948 'Eugenic Protection Law' that legalised forced sterilisation of the mentally ill and those with hereditary diseases; however the issue was complicated by the inclusion in the same bill of legalisation of abortion on grounds of 'economic hardship', which became the focus of interest of women's rights groups looking to strengthen women's reproductive rights. This divergence of interest groups meant that the use of international forums by pro-rights groups became crucial in leading to the replacement of the Eugenic Protection Law by the Maternal Body Protection Law in 1996. In the last case, satisfactory resolution still remains unreached (Amnesty International 2011).

A further example is provided in the exploration by Tsutsui and Shin (2008) of the position regarding the human rights of Koreans resident in Japan. In this case global human rights norms provided vocabularies that helped to construct cohesive activism within the country, and proved a more successful basis to argue for change than a basis in citizenship rights. International forums and pressure from outside Japan, from networks of international human rights activists, also created pressure on the Japanese government, contributing to successful change within Japan. Holland's examination of role of the Japanese Supreme Court (Holland 2009: 79) finds it to be a 'timid and largely deferential institution', acting as a brake on the lower courts whenever judges attempt to challenge a law or action on human rights grounds, and largely upholding government policies that are being challenged on rights grounds. He argues that this has led to the development of rights-oriented NGOs within Japan, and the use of human rights defenders. Holland (2009) does however find signs that the stance of the Supreme Court may change in the future, consequent on pressures on Japan's leadership role within the region, and the arrival of a new generation of lawyers in the Supreme Court, as well as increasing international pressure on its human rights policies.

Linking national human rights institutions into the UN system

At the International Conference held in Tunis in 1993, NHRIs established the International Coordinating Committee of NHRIs (ICC) to help coordinate the activities of the NHRI network. In 1998, rules of procedures were developed for the ICC and its membership was enlarged to sixteen members, four from each of the geographical regions. At that same meeting, the ICC resolved to create a process

Table 4.3 Members of the Bureau of the ICC and Regional Coordinating bodies

Bureau members
- The New Zealand Human Rights Commission (ICC Chair) http://www.hrc.co.nz
- Kenya National Commission on Human Rights (ICC Secretary) http://www.knchr.org/
- The Conseil Consultatif des Droits de L'Homme du Maroc http://www.ccdh.org.ma Chair of the African Network of NHRIs
- South African Human Rights Commission http://www.sahrc.org.za/
- National Commission for Human Rights of Togo http://www.cndh-togo.org
- Comisión Nacional para los Derechos Humanos of Mexico http://www.cndh.org.mx
- Ombudsman of Ecuador http://www.dlh.lahora.com.ec/paginas/judicial/PAGINAS/Defensoria.base.htm Chair of the NHRIs in the Americas
- Procuraduria de Defensa de los Derechos Humanos of El Salvador
- Defensoría del Pueblo de la Nación Argentina http://www.defensor.gov.ar
- Australian Human Rights Commission http://www.hreoc.gov.au/ Chair of the Asia Pacific Network of NHRIs
- National Human Rights Commission of India http://nhrc.nic.in
- National Centre for Human Rights of Jordan http://www.nchr.org.jo/
- Irish Human Rights Commission http://www.ihrc.ie/home/default.asp Chair of the European Group of NHRIs
- Commission consultative des droits de l'homme of Luxembourg http://www.ccdh.lu
- German Institute for Human Rights http://www.institut-fuer-menschenrechte.de
- The Office of the Ombudsman of Croatia http://www.ombudsman.hr/

Regional Coordinating bodies
- Africa: Permanent Secretariat of the Network of African NHRIs http://www.nanhri.org/
- Americas: Network of the NHRIs of the Americas http://www.rindhca.org.ve/?idiomaSeleccion=ing (much of text in Spanish)
- Asia-Pacific: Asia-Pacific Forum http://www.asiapacificforum.net/
- Europe: European Group of NHRIs http://www.ihrc.ie/international/euronhrigroups.html

for accrediting institutions. In 2008, the ICC discussed governance issues, including incorporation of the ICC in order to better cope with the changing environment, including the developing role of NHRIs in the international human rights system. The ICC decided to incorporate itself as a legal entity under Swiss law, with a bureau of sixteen voting members representing the four regions of the ICC ('A status' NHRIs, see Table 4.3).

The ICC also decided to streamline rules of procedures and to clearly define its membership and the role and governance of its annual meeting and international conferences. In 2009, the ICC discussed matters related to the Committee's governance working group and the working group on sustainable funding and the Subcommittee on Accreditation. General Meetings of the ICC, meetings of the ICC Bureau and of the Subcommittee on Accreditation, as well as International Conferences of the ICC, are held under the auspices of, and in cooperation with, OHCHR. The ICC links NHRIs directly into the UN system. The accreditation system governs access to UN committees. Institutions accredited by the ICC with 'A status', meaning full compliance with the Paris Principles, are usually accorded speaking rights and seating at human rights treaty bodies and other UN organs. The

ICC representative often presents statements on behalf of individual NHRIs or the regional groups.

The ICC has one member of staff representing it at the United Nations Office at Geneva. Secretariat support is provided to the ICC by the National Institutions and Regional Mechanisms (NIRM) Unit of the Field Operations and Technical Cooperation Division of the Office of the United Nations High Commissioner for Human Rights (OHCHR). Additional work devolves on the NHRI elected to chair the network, currently the New Zealand Human Rights Commission, and the chairs of the ICC's four regional networks. The peer review process for initial accreditation, and reaccreditation every five years, is managed by a subcommittee consisting of one representative of each of the regional networks. The ICC holds annual general meetings (usually in Geneva in March, coinciding with the UN Human Rights Council session) and a biennial thematic conference.

The National Human Rights Institutions Forum is a web portal maintained on behalf of the ICC by the OHCHR. As at May 2011, it shows a list of 126 national institutions. Of those, sixty-seven are currently accredited with 'A status' by the ICC, and are thus entitled to vote or hold office in the ICC or its regional groups, fifteen are partially compliant with the Paris Principles (B status), seven are non-compliant and thirty-six have not yet been assessed.

The Asia-Pacific Forum of National Human Rights Institutions (APF) is the largest (in terms of number of members – national human rights institutions that comply with the Paris Principles) regional human rights organisation in the Asia-Pacific. It was established in 1996 to support the establishment and strengthening of national human rights institutions in the region. Current members are national institutions in fifteen different countries across the Asia-Pacific region: Afghanistan, Australia, India, Indonesia, Jordan, Malaysia, Mongolia, Nepal, New Zealand, Palestine Territories, Philippines, Qatar, Republic of Korea, Thailand and Timor-Leste. The APF provides a framework for national human rights institutions to work together and cooperate on a regional basis through a wide range of services, including training, capacity building, networks and staff exchanges.

According to the latest report on the Universal Periodic Review for Sweden (HRCl 2010), Sweden is considering the establishment of an independent national human rights institution. The agency represented by the Equality Ombudsman, discussed above, is not accredited by the ICC (FRA 2010c), although the predecessor Ombudsman for Equal Rights did have A status accreditation which lapsed at the end of 2008 (FRA 2010c). Ghana's CHRAJ is accorded A status by the ICC, as is Australia's HREOC and India's NHRC. Japan has no NHRI listed on the ICC system.

Later treaties in the UN human rights system have been formulated with an explicit role for NHRIs in their implementation or monitoring, namely the Optional Protocol to the Convention Against Torture (OPCAT), which entered into force in June 2006 and the Convention on the Rights of Persons with Disabilities (CRPD), which entered into force in May 2008. Pohjolainen (2006) sees this as a return of an idea circulating in the earliest years of the UN that national committees should be established to monitor compliance with the UDHR.

Protecting and promoting human rights: how successful are national human rights systems?

The examples of the different countries considered above demonstrate the variety that exists in structure, organisation, mandate and functioning of the different national human rights systems. Given the variety that exists, and the highly diverse economic and socio-political contexts pertaining in different countries, it should come as no surprise that there is considerable variation in terms of achievements of the different systems in terms of protecting and promoting human rights within countries.

One factor worthy of consideration is the question of whether at country level a single or multiple human rights institutions is to be preferred. Carver (2011) provides a recent analysis, identifying that there is no guidance on this point within international and regional human rights standards. The Paris Principles (OHCHR 1993) give no explicit guidance, although they do state that an NHRI should 'be given as broad a mandate as possible' (OHCHR 1993: para 2). After a detailed consideration of the arguments both for and against single institutions, Carver (2011) concludes that arguments of both pragmatism and effectiveness are 'overwhelmingly' in favour of a single institution, noting that a number of countries have at different times decided in favour of a merger of different national institutions, Australia (in 1986), the UK (in 2006) and Sweden (in 2008). Not all countries have chosen to do this however. Hungary maintains four separate, but connected, ombudsman institutions, and Lithuania has three ombudsman institutions which operate almost entirely separately (Carver 2011).

As can be seen from the sections above on individual countries, the outcomes from the different national systems are extremely varied, and direct comparison is impossible given the many and diverse factors affecting achievement, including resourcing, timelines, simplicity or access to proceedings, but also the variation in socio-political context. Elsewhere, in the research literature, some studies have examined what has been achieved within national systems broadly, and particularly in relation to the right to health. The case study summarises some mixed evidence obtained in an examination of one part of the UK's human rights system. As Finnegan et al. (2010) point out, the United States has maintained an ambivalent relationship with the discourse of international human rights. In particular, the United States has ratified less than a third of the international human rights instruments. Finnegan et al. (2010) explore how US human rights activists conceptualise, relate to and utilise the human rights framework, finding that activists contend with substantial political obstacles, including the US government's perceived exploitations of the human rights framework. Activists considered that deep-seated American cultural identities of liberalism, meritocracy and exceptionalism acted as strong barriers to the use of a human rights framework, however they still saw grassroots approaches as a potential avenue for future human rights organising in the US context.

A review by Hogerzeil et al. (2006) examined completed court cases in low- and middle-income countries where individuals or groups had sought access to essential medicines, with reference to the right to health. The review identified successful

Case study: The effectiveness of the UK's Joint Committee on Human Rights

In 2001, the UK parliament created the Joint Committee on Human Rights (JCHR) to scrutinise legislation for compliance with the UK's 1998 Human Rights Act and the UK's international human rights commitments. This is an example of a 'Commonwealth model of constitutionalism', where parliament and parliamentary committees are seen as lead agents in promoting and safeguarding rights, in contrast to the American model where judicial review and the courts are seen as the main route for rights protection. The JCHR's responsibilities include: first, reviewing proposed new bills for rights problems during the drafting and passage of new legislation; secondly, reviewing remedial orders following a domestic court's issuance of a 'declaration of incompatibility' or an adverse judgment by the ECHR. Examining the achievements of the JCHR in a variety of ways presents a mixed picture with regard to their influence:

- a very low percentage of the bills scrutinised over the period from its creation until 2005 were modified as a result of the JCHR (3 per cent);
- the JCHR had achieved a high level of awareness of its reports on prospective bills in its first five years;
- in terms of its monitoring function, out of the eighteen declarations of incompatibility made by the courts up to the end of 2005, twelve are still standing and the JCHR did not report on the six where the legislation has been changed;
- in terms of the Counter-Terrorism Bill, the JCHR issued six reports, particularly criticising the government's proposal to increase to forty-two the number of days suspected terrorists may be detained without charge. The government proceeded with the bill, and it was passed in the House of Commons in June 2008. The JCHR's reports did however influence the debate on the bill, and it was initially defeated in the House of Lords, and only passed into legislation once the increase in pre-charge detention was removed.

(Summarised from Tolley 2009)

cases in ten countries, eight countries in Central and Latin America, plus India and South Africa. Their interpretation of their findings is that litigation can help ensure that governments fulfil their human rights obligations in this respect, but they suggest that the courts should be used as a last resort and that it is better to ensure that human rights considerations are planned into policy and programmes. The review by Singh *et al.* (2007) highlights positive health reforms that have been achieved in four different countries, Argentina, Ecuador, South Africa and India, by use of legal measures; they identify four factors as responsible for the extensive successes in South Africa and India: intense and sustained pressure by strong and competent civil society organisations in those countries; fairly independent, competent and progressive judicial authorities; governments having respect for the rule of law; and use of medical evidence to support legal arguments.

Looking specifically at the right to health, the South East Asian Regional Office of WHO has summarised the positioning of the right to health in the constitutions of the eleven countries contained in this WHO region (SEARO 2011), finding the right positively stated in six of the countries (DPR Korea, Indonesia, Maldives, Nepal, Thailand and Timor-Leste), while the other five countries (Bhutan, Bangladesh, India, Myanmar and Sri Lanka) do not explicitly state this as a positive right but nonetheless compel the state to provide health services and in some cases to improve public health (SEARO 2011). However, as has been discussed in the section on India earlier in this chapter, lack of statement of a positive right to health in the constitution has not prevented this right being inferred from others that are constitutionally mandated. Presence of the right to health in the constitution is, also, a long way from a guarantee that the right will be implemented. Finally, and most comprehensively of all, Backman *et al.* (2008) propose seventy-two indicators that reflect some of the health system features associated with the right to health and uses globally processed data on these indicators for 194 countries as well as national data for five other countries to assess the state of achievement of the right to health, finding a very mixed picture of achievement.

As yet, there is no comprehensive overview of the functioning and effectiveness of national systems and NHRIs. A set of benchmarks and indicators has been produced (ICHRP 2005), but these have not yet been taken up in a comprehensive fashion. Some are reflected in the OHCHR survey on NHRIs mentioned at the beginning of the chapter (OHCHR 2009a) which provides some insight into the factors that NHRIs themselves consider impinge on their effectiveness. Factors identified include: limited capacity to follow up on recommendations, a particular issue in Africa and the Americas; lack of diversity in the composition of governing bodies; lack of sufficient resources or materials to carry out human rights education and research in many cases where there was the mandate to carry out this function; and finally, the need to strengthen relationships with relevant national stakeholders, particularly public bodies such as the executive, parliament and the judiciary.

Within the European Union, the European Agency for Fundamental Rights (FRA) has recently published a report on NHRIs in the EU Member States (FRA 2010c), intended to identify gaps and concerns in what it calls the fundamental rights architecture of the EU, looking at data protection bodies, equality bodies and NHRIs. This identifies that in many of the EU member states without an NHRI fully compliant with the Paris Principles (currently seventeen of the twenty-seven member states), human rights education and awareness-raising, promotion of human rights and interaction with civil society are either not mandated, or not carried out due to resource constraints. Their report recommends that the Paris Principles should be seen as the very minimum standards for NHRIs in the European Union.

Perhaps it is not surprising that the picture given of the performance and achievements of national human rights systems is somewhat patchy, given that in many countries the NHRIs concerned, if they exist, are relatively young. As has already been noted, an increasing role may be played by these institutions in terms of monitoring human rights compliance at country level. The deliberations on strengthening human rights systems initiated by the current High Commissioner for Human Rights may well provide for an increased role for NHRIs in the future.

5 Human rights and health equity

The links between health and human rights

In terms of understanding the links between health and human rights it is useful to distinguish three different, but interacting, components (WHO 2002a). First, human rights violations can directly affect health: for example, torture, slavery, violence against women and children and harmful traditional practices. Secondly, the promotion of human rights, in particular those connected to the social determinants of health, for example rights to education, to food and nutrition, shelter and employment, lead to reduced vulnerability to ill health and promote health. Thirdly, health development can involve promotion or violation of human rights depending on how it affects rights such as the right to participation, freedom from discrimination, right to information and right to privacy. There is a reciprocal impact of health and human rights. The promotion, protection, restriction or violations of human rights have direct and indirect impacts on health and wellbeing, in the short, medium and long term.

In terms of illustrating the strong links between health equity and human rights, the intersection between HIV positivity and drug use provides an excellent example; others are given in the two case studies in this chapter, the first on domestic violence and the second on indigenous rights. Jürgens *et al.* (2010) summarise the considerable evidence on the link between human rights abuses experienced by people who use drugs and vulnerability to HIV infection and access to services. Their review summarises a wide range of studies on people who use drugs, demonstrating not only widespread abuses of human rights, but also that these occur in ways that increase vulnerability to HIV infection, and negatively affect delivery of HIV services. The abuses identified include denial of harm-reduction services, discriminatory access to antiretroviral therapy, abusive law enforcement practices and coercive treatment for drug dependence. Jürgens *et al.* (2010) argue therefore that protection of the human rights of people who use drugs is important not only because of their human rights, but also because it is an essential precondition to improving their health.

Sarin *et al.* (2011) also illustrate the direct effects of human rights violations on health, through a study of injecting drug users in Delhi, India. Their study identifies many human rights abuses experienced, including denial of access to

Case study: Domestic violence: a major public health and human rights issue

Domestic violence, abuse against women or men by current or previous intimate partners, is a major public health problem globally (Garcia-Moreno *et al.* 2005). It occurs in all countries irrespective of culture, socio-economic status or religion, and in all types of relationships, both same-sex and heterosexual (Krug *et al.* 2002). The context and severity of violence by men against women makes domestic violence against women a much larger problem in public health terms (Krug *et al.* 2002; WHO 1997). Intimate partner abuse has severe short- and long-term health consequences, both physical and mental, for the partner experiencing abuse and for any children in the family (Itzin *et al.* 2010a).

A frequent characteristic of domestic violence is that the perpetrator often blames his abuse on the woman and her behaviour, and uses the abuse to assert control over the woman and her life. The woman experiencing abuse is often made to feel inadequate, a failure, and that she deserves the abuse. Sometimes her movements are curtailed and she is kept a virtual prisoner in the house. These characteristics have led to domestic violence being viewed legally as a human rights issue (Chapman 1990), and to cases being brought under the UN and regional systems for the protection of human rights.

One of the earliest was in 1998, when a petition was presented to the Inter-American Commission on Human Rights (IACHR) bringing the case of a Brazilian woman, Maria da Penha, who had suffered years of abuse from her husband. Despite numerous reports to various authorities within the country, no action was taken. As UN Women (2011: 18) documents, in 2006, the Government of Brazil enacted domestic violence legislation, symbolically named the Maria da Penha Law on domestic and family violence, mandating preventative measures, special courts and tough sentences. Two further cases were brought by NGOs against Austria, on behalf of two women murdered by their husbands, to the CEDAW Committee under the Optional Protocol. The Committee's decisions on the cases in 2007 were of global significance because they made clear that the state's obligation to protect women from domestic violence extends beyond passing laws. The Committee found that Austria had failed to act with 'due diligence', by not ensuring that the law was implemented properly. In response to the Committee's recommendations and the media attention that surrounded the case, the Austrian government introduced and accelerated legal reforms to protect women from violence (UN Women 2011: 18).

For a further example of the value of a human rights framework in domestic violence, this time in addressing a different range of social and cultural factors that come into play in the case of refugee women in Australia who experience domestic violence, see the paper by Rees (2004).

health services, arrests and physical and verbal abuse. They find a strong association between suicidal ideation and human rights abuses, with the likelihood of suicidal ideation being strongly related to the cumulative amount of abuse experienced. Wolfe and Malinowska-Sempruch (2007) also examine how conflicting drug policies have had a wide range of human rights implications. They explore how harm-reduction approaches to drug users, which include needle exchanges and methadone maintenance programmes, despite proving effective in trials from countries as diverse as Australia, Belarus and Thailand, are still not welcomed in many countries with rapid growth in HIV through injecting drug users, who continue to prefer policies based on criminal enforcement and demands for abstinence. They identify the challenges caused by the UN drug conventions which sit uneasily with approaches that are based on harm minimisation and or human rights, and emphasise the importance of advocacy by countries which are implementing harm minimisation strategies and the need for NGOs to press for the adoption of effective and rights-based policies. The current special rapporteur on the right to health, Anand Grover, argued, in a report (Grover 2010) prepared for discussion at the sixty-fifth session of the UN General Assembly, that the current international system of drug control, based on law enforcement policies and criminal sanctions, has failed. Instead, he argues that a harm-reduction approach, set within a right to health approach, is needed to ensure that the rights of people who use drugs are respected, protected and fulfilled.

Given this understanding of the close interrelationships between health equity and human rights, it is obviously desirable to ensure that health policies and programmes protect and promote rights. This has led for calls for the use of rights-based approaches (RBA) in policy development and implementation and in the planning and delivery of health programmes, understanding RBA to mean approaches that help protect and promote rights. Accepting health equity as a goal of health systems worldwide thus necessitates a focus on human rights, and indeed vice versa. This chapter sets out to explore in more detail what can be meant by the term 'rights-based approach' and how effective this can be in moving towards health equity and social justice. The next chapter then deals with the question of how the human rights implications of existing or planned policies and programmes can be explored.

Rights-based approaches to health policy and practice

The first thing to consider is what exactly should be understood by a rights-based approach to health. According to WHO (2002a) this has three components, it refers to the processes of: using human rights as a framework for health development; assessing and addressing the human rights implications of any health policy, programme or legislation; and making human rights an integral dimension of the design, implementation, monitoring and evaluation of health-related policies and programmes in *all* spheres, including political, economic and social. Singh (2010) identifies four key features or principles of RBAs: the realisation of rights without discrimination; the principle of accountability to rights-holders by duty-bearers;

Case study: Health of indigenous Australians: the importance of protecting and promoting rights

The health status of indigenous Australians is shaped by the legacy of centuries of social disadvantage, dispossession, discrimination and colonialism. The current position is still characterised by social disadvantage in many areas including education, housing, employment and income. Life expectancy (ABS 2009) of indigenous men is 67.2 (compared to non-indigenous men 78.7) and of indigenous women is 72.9 (compared to non-indigenous 82.6).

In 2007, in response to the report of an inquiry into child sexual abuse in indigenous communities in the Northern Territory (Wild and Anderson 2007), the Australian Commonwealth government introduced the Northern Territory Emergency Response (NTER), a package of eleven emergency measures including compulsory child health checks and significant welfare reforms. Legislation was introduced to do this and provisions in three of the acts were deemed to be 'special measures', allowing the suspension of part of the Racial Discrimination Act. There was much concern about this, about many aspects of the processes through which the NTER was developed and implemented, and about some of its major provisions, including the use of the army to lead implementation, the acquiring of land title in prescribed communities, compulsory income management for all adults in prescribed communities who were receiving welfare payments and compulsory health checks for children. In addition the measures in the NTER were not well matched with the recommendations from the inquiry itself.

An independent review of the NTER measures was set up by the Australian government in June 2008, involving consultation with those affected by the measures. The review's overarching recommendations (NTER Review Board) were:

- that the Federal and Northern Territory Governments recognise as a matter of urgent national significance the continuing need to address the unacceptably high level of disadvantage and social dislocation being experienced by Aboriginal Australians living in remote communities throughout the Northern Territory;
- in addressing these needs both governments acknowledge the requirement to reset their relationship with indigenous people based on genuine consultation, engagement and partnership;
- that government actions affecting indigenous communities respect Australia's human rights obligations and conform with the Racial Discrimination Act 1975.

The Australian government accepted the review's overarching recommendations and commenced action to give effect to them. In June 2010, the Parliament passed legislation to reinstate the Racial Discrimination Act 1975 in relation to the NTER and make necessary changes to the NTER laws.

A health impact assessment of the NTER was undertaken, with a human rights component, by the Australian Indigenous Doctors' Association (AIDA) in collaboration with the Centre for Health Equity Training, Research and Evaluation at the University of New South Wales (CHETRE). This began in late 2007 and the full report was published in 2010 (AIDA and CHETRE 2010). The assessment concludes:

> the intended health outcomes of the NTER (improved health and wellbeing, and ultimately, life expectancy) are unlikely to be fully achieved. It is predicted that it will leave a negative legacy on the psychological and social wellbeing, on the spirituality and cultural integrity of the prescribed communities. However, it may be possible to minimise or mitigate these negative impacts if the Australian and Northern Territory governments commit to and invest in taking the steps necessary to work in respectful partnership with the Aboriginal leaders and organisations responsible for the governance of the prescribed communities in the NT. The principal recommendations arising from the HIA are based on the evidence (from communities, stakeholders and experts) that it is essential to find ways to work together as equals.
>
> (AIDA and CHETRE 2010: 55)

There is ongoing debate as to whether the Australian government's response has fully taken on board all the points raised and debate continues. See for example papers within the Universal Periodic Review of Australia in 2011 on the OHCHR website and Harris and Gartland (2011).

a recognition of the importance of participation in process; and finally adaptation to the local context. An expansion of these in the context of a human rights-based approach to development programming is provided by Silva (2003) reporting on the common understanding achieved among the different UN agencies working in the field, although some have criticised this. For example, Gruskin et al. (2010: 134) refer to it as 'a lowest common denominator approach'. Nyamu-Musembi and Cornwall (2004), in their review of the different methodologies associated with RBAs in the field of development, argue that RBAs would mean little if they have no potential to achieve a positive transformation of power relations among the various development actors. Berman (2008), again focusing on development projects, provides a succinct summary of principles in the acronym PANEL (participation, accountability, non-discrimination and equality, empowerment and linkages to human rights standards). WHO (2002a) provides a slightly longer mnemonic summarising the possible ingredients of a rights-based approach to health (see Table 5.1). Finally, Gruskin et al.

Table 5.1 Possible 'ingredients' in a rights-based approach to health

Right to health
Information
Gender
Human dignity
Transparency
Siracusa principles
Benchmarks and indicators
Accountability
Safeguards
Equality and freedom from discrimination
Disaggregation
Attention to vulnerable groups
Participation
Privacy
Right to education
Optimal balance between public health goals and protection of human rights
Accessibility
Concrete government obligations
Human rights expressly linked

Source: WHO 2002a: 17

(2010) offer a four-question framework for assessing RBAs to health (with a further set of at least four questions embedded in one of the questions); most importantly, they draw attention to a minimum list of principles that must be included: participation; non-discrimination; service availability, accessibility, acceptability and quality; transparency and accountability.

The past thirty years have seen the development of a wealth of different approaches and assessment tools for assisting in the task of ensuring that health policies and programmes respect, protect and promote human rights. Worm (2010) in a recent review examines no fewer than seventeen different approaches to impact assessment in the field of human rights and gender equality, although not all of these explicitly draw on international human rights standards in their conceptual frameworks. In the remainder of this chapter the use of rights-based approaches is discussed by means of a range of different examples concerned with changing policy and/or practice. They are organised into four different sections. The first looks at policy advocacy and considers several different chapters in the history of response to the challenge of HIV/AIDS where rights-based argumentation has been influential in driving forward change. The second section focuses on rights-based approaches to programme planning, and examines the work of CARE International. The third section turns to practice in individual care and considers rights-based approaches in individual interactions between health/welfare professionals and patients/clients. The fourth section examines human rights education, focusing in particular on rights-based rights education as empowerment education. The chapter concludes with a brief reflection on the current state of the growing RBA industry.

Policy advocacy

The earliest significant body of work using rights-based approaches for health policy advocacy purposes was in the field of HIV/AIDS, where the work carried out demonstrated the power of rights-based argumentation in securing appropriate treatment and resources for people living with HIV/AIDS. Later in this section, some of the chapters from this history are examined, exploring action taken to seek improved access to essential medicines, and ARVs in particular.

The various human rights treaties clearly assign governments the role of ensuring the right to health, and discussions on the right to health are often implicitly based on an assumption that the government is the sole or major provider of health services, or at least that services reside in the not-for-profit sector. Apart from attention to the pharmaceutical industry and action to try and improve access to essential medicines, very little attention has been given to the role of for-profit enterprise in the realisation of the right to health. One exception is McBeth (2004) who considers what happens to the state's human rights duties when services are privatised. Considering three specific areas where this experience is common, health, education and prisons, he argues that such private providers of social services have human rights obligations and, at the same time, the state's obligations change in nature from a duty of action to one of supervision, and if necessary intervention. Another exception is the paper by Kinney (2010) who examines how for-profit enterprise has worked at cross purposes with the achievement of the right to health, and explores a number of principles that might assist private for-profit enterprises in adopting a supportive role.

A further example of rights-based policy advocacy is provided by De Negri Filho (2008). Drawing on work on Latin American social medicine in Brazil, Colombia and Venezuela, he discusses new ways of thinking about social fragility (instead of risks) and developing inter-sectoral programming to improve care, as well as to reduce inequalities among population groups. The article argues that a rights-based approach can be a concrete tool for restructuring both public policies and action.

Donald and Mottershaw (2009) carried out an analysis, commissioned by the UK's NHRI (the Equality and Human Rights Commission), of cases brought to court under the UK's Human Rights Act, which came into force in 2000, or the European Convention on Human Rights. They were concerned to examine the impact on policy and practice among public authorities in England and Wales. The UK's Human Rights Act provides for cases of breach of the European Convention to be heard in UK courts and made it unlawful for a public authority, such as government departments, local authorities or the police, to act in a way that is incompatible with a Convention right. They analysed ten selected cases, all of which involved civil and political rights, and several of which also involved economic and social rights, through addressing health, housing or destitution. They used a range of methods to trace the impact of the decisions on policy and practice; a detailed analysis of each case can be found in Donald *et al.* (2009). Their paper finds some, but limited, evidence of direct impact on policy and practice; however, they note the methodological difficulties of establishing this. They argue that one factor hindering impact was the absence of a body like the Equality and Human Rights Commission, which only came into being in 2007, and which might draw out the implications of court cases for policy and practice and promote the necessary changes. They identify a particularly significant role for advocacy from service users and advocacy organisations.

HIV/AIDS: struggles over access to essential medicines

As an exploration of the role of rights-based approaches in health policy, this section looks at a couple of distinct chapters in the history of the global response to HIV/AIDS, and in particular at the issue of trying to ensure access to essential medicines. The '3 by 5' initiative, launched by UNAIDS and WHO in 2003 (WHO/UNAIDS 2006), set a global target of providing 3 million people living with HIV/AIDS in low- and middle-income countries with life-prolonging antiretroviral treatment (ARV) by the end of 2005. This was one step towards the goal of ensuring universal access to HIV/AIDS prevention and treatment. According to the UNAIDS/WHO '3 by 5' progress report in 2006, although the target was not reached, with around 1.3 million people living with HIV receiving ARV therapy in low- and middle-income countries, 20 per cent of those in need of treatment were receiving it. More impressively, the number of people receiving antiretroviral treatment in low- and middle-income countries increased over fivefold from the end of 2001 to 2005 (WHO/UNAIDS 2006). What was behind this? One part of the answer lies in human rights argumentation, and its interaction with intellectual property law, and this provides a good example of the effectiveness of a rights-based approach to health at the global, international level.

Key players in this story are the multinational drug companies (Lage 2011). In most low-income countries access to imported drugs is heavily limited by their expense, which is maintained by patent law in the country of origin of the drug patent. Domestic production in low-income countries is limited by the ability to create a domestic industry, something that has been achieved in relatively few low-income countries; exceptions include Brazil and India, and the positive effects of these will be considered later. Fear of growth in domestic production, combined with World Trade Organization (WTO) moves towards harmonisation in trade, led to moves to extend or modify patent laws in low-income countries. These moves caused great public health concern as the introduction of process and product patents on drugs would be likely to decrease access to drugs to a significant extent, through three different mechanisms: abrupt rises in prices; deleterious impacts on local pharmaceutical industries; and a greater emphasis on private-sector research and development (Cullet 2003).

Patents (and patent law) protect intellectual property rights, so a relevant question becomes: do intellectual property rights qualify as human rights? While the short answer is a resounding *no*, the arguments as to why are important to understand. The debates of 1948 and 1957 indicate that the basic human rights treaties did NOT intend to recognise the interests of authors or inventors as fundamental human rights (Sub-Commission on the Promotion and Protection of Human Rights 2001). Instead, both the Universal Declaration of Human Rights and the International Covenant on Economic, Social and Cultural Rights recognise as a basic claim *everyone's* right to enjoy the fruits of cultural life and scientific development and the right of the individual author is subsidiary in the balancing of priorities; the implication is that human rights put the emphasis on societal benefits, a communitarian approach (Sub-Commission on the Promotion and Protection of Human Rights 2001). Thus intellectual property rights are *temporary* and can be *revoked* and *transferred*, while human rights are *inalienable* and *timeless* (CESCR 2001). This provides an important opening for human rights-based argumentation in connection with patent laws.

Moving on, 1994 saw the introduction of the World Trade Organization (WTO) TRIPS (Trade-Related Aspects of Intellectual Property Rights) agreement. TRIPS sought to provide minimum levels of intellectual property protection in all WTO member states ('t Hoen 2005). A key clause of the TRIPS agreement provided that intellectual property rights should 'contribute to the promotion of technological innovation and to the transfer and dissemination of technology' (article 7). Implementation of this provision requires a certain level of flexibility that can be useful, and this was deliberate following the understanding that human rights did not include intellectual property rights for the individual.

The agreement also includes, importantly, the provision that states can adopt measures necessary to protect *public health* and to promote the *public interest* in sectors of vital importance to their socio-economic and technological development (article 8). The multinational pharmaceutical industry has been concerned about the implication of TRIPS for their profits. Here some episodes in this (continuing) history are considered, the first in relation to South Africa, and the second Brazil.

In 1997 the South African Medicines and Related Substances Control Amendment Act was introduced; this aimed to increase the availability of affordable medicines via provisions including generic substitution of off-patent medicine, transparent pricing for all medicines and the parallel importing of patented medicines (Fisher and Rigamonti 2005). This was challenged in the South African High Court, in a case filed in 1998 by a consortium of pharmaceutical companies; their challenge was on the basis that the act amounted to a violation of TRIPS and of the South African constitution. The nub of the argument to be considered in the Court was whether South Africa was misusing the flexibilities within TRIPS.

Before the case came to court, a dirty fight started aiming to influence the outcome in the pharmaceutical companies' favour. The US put pressure on South Africa by withholding trade benefits and threatening further trade sanctions. AIDS activists in the US then entered the fray, on the side of increased access to medicines, and as a result of increasing public pressure the US changed its stance by the end of 1999 ('t Hoen 2005). In 2000, the case began to be heard by South African High Court (case no. 4183/98). By this point, public opinion was now against the position of the pharmaceutical companies on a widespread basis. Several governments and the European Parliament demanded that the companies should withdraw; they eventually unconditionally did so in April 2001 (Fisher and Rigamonti 2005).

These events raised two important issues. First, the interpretation of the flexibilities of TRIPS and their use for public health purposes needed clarification if low-income countries were to be able to use the provisions without threat of legal or political challenges. Secondly, it became clear that high-income countries that exercised trade pressures to defend the interests of their multinational industries needed to recognise that this would result in counter-pressure being exerted by NGOs and public health/human rights activists ('t Hoen 2005).

Turning now to a second episode, the case of US versus Brazil is considered. Beginning in the mid-1990s, Brazil offered comprehensive AIDS care including universal access to ARV treatment; this programme succeeded in reducing AIDS-related mortality and morbidity dramatically from the late 1990s (Nunn *et al.* 2009). One reason behind this success was Brazil's ability to produce medicines locally, with generic competition resulting in reductions in prices of ARV and lower prices for patented drugs being negotiated using threat of production under compulsory licence, a possibility created by article 68 of the Brazilian patent law, which allows a patent to be used *without* the consent of the patent holder. Additionally Brazil offered a cooperation agreement including technology transfer to low-income countries for the production of generic ARV drugs ('t Hoen 2005). In February 2001, the US took action against Brazil at the WTO Dispute Settlement Body, arguing that article 68 discriminated against US owners of Brazilian patents and that it curtailed patent holders' rights and was in violation of TRIPS articles. The US action came under immediate and fierce pressure from the international NGO community, and some five months later, in June 2001, the US withdrew ('t Hoen 2005). Later chapters in the struggle for essential medicines and Brazil's pivotal role in this are covered by Nunn *et al.* (2009).

In both these examples, NGOs played a key role in advancing human rights argumentation and drawing attention to the flexibilities potentially available within TRIPS (e.g. see www.msfaccess.org: this website, run by MSF's Campaign for Access to Essential Medicines, is an excellent source of information on the ongoing struggles in both courts and policy arena to ensure access to medicines globally). But there were other players that were also important.

First, the public health community: the 1996 World Health Assembly passed a resolution requesting WHO to report on the impact of WTO's work with respect to national drug policies and essential drugs and make recommendations for collaboration between WTO and WHO as appropriate. Very importantly, this gave WHO the mandate to produce a guide to implementing TRIPS while limiting the negative effects of higher patent protection on drug availability. This was published in 1998. The United States and a number of European countries unsuccessfully pressured WHO in an attempt to stop publication, and the European Director-General for Trade of the European Commission stated: 'No priority should be given to health over intellectual property considerations' (DG1 1998: 1). Fortunately, this stance was not allowed to prevail ('t Hoen 2005). Since then WHO has adopted progressively stronger resolutions in the area, and the issue has also been taken up in various positive ways by other international organisations, including the UN Sub-Commission for Promotion and Protection of Human Rights (superseded by the Human Rights Council in 2006), UNDP, EU, UNAIDS, World Bank and OAU.

The 2001 fourth WTO Ministerial Conference saw the Doha Declaration on TRIPS and public health, including the following very important article 4:

> We agree that the TRIPS Agreement does not and should not prevent Members from taking measures to protect public health. Accordingly, while reiterating our commitment to the TRIPS Agreement, we affirm that the Agreement can and should be interpreted and implemented in a manner supportive of WTO Members' right to protect public health and, in particular, to promote access to medicines for all.

This can be seen as providing confirmation that public health concerns outweigh full protection of intellectual property. Whether this represents a temporary or permanent victory still remains to be seen. Struggles still go on and reports continue to appear of industrialised countries offering technical assistance to developing countries in drafting new patent laws that in fact do not use TRIPS flexibilities fully and support instead the interests of the pharmaceutical companies. As the Access to Medicines campaign emphasises, there is still a need for vigilance.

As a final episode taken from the story of RBAs in responding to the challenge of HIV/AIDS, the case of South Africa's Treatment Action Campaign (TAC) provides an excellent example of the possibilities realised by combining law and social mobilisation in support of the right to health. Heywood (2009) provides a fascinating analysis of the history of the first ten years of TAC from its beginnings with a small demonstration in support of the right to treatment on International Human Rights Day in December 1998. TAC is primarily a member-/volunteer-based organisation (Heywood 2009), and has always sought active links with other mass-based organisations within South African civil society, including churches and trade unions. It is organised and operates at local (community), provincial and national level. Starting with no paid staff or budget, after ten years TAC had over 100 staff and a budget of US$5 million in 2007.

As well as contributing to the struggles against the pharmaceutical industry described above, TAC's successes include achieving successful constitutional litigation for a national programme to prevent mother to child transmission of HIV (2001–2), access to the implementation plan for ARV rollout (2004) and access to ARV treatment for prisoners at Westville prison in KwaZulu Natal province (2006–7). Finally Heywood traces their success in achieving price reductions for ARVs and other medicines, and achieving more equitable funding for services for HIV/AIDS and STIs. He notes, importantly, that this example identifies clearly the value of the use of both litigation and social mobilisation in combination with one another, arguing that it would be a mistake to rely on just one of these alone. Gauri et al. (2007) describe in detail how adopting a rights-based approach in relation to HIV/AIDS in Brazil led to the wider demand for universal access to health care for all Brazilian citizens. They present a detailed analysis of the period from the early 1980s to 2003, showing the important contributions of social mobilisation around HIV/AIDS and of key NGOs; non-discrimination and the right to health care were key principles, and legislation supporting these was part of the response.

Rights-based approaches to programme planning

This section turns to an examination of programme planning using RBAs. There are a number of manuals and tool kits. Jonsson (2003) describes UNICEF's rights-based approach to development programming, and Chopra and Ford (2005) consider a human rights approach to health promotion, drawing on the UNICEF approach. A resource pack has also been produced by ActionAid International in collaboration with a number of NGOs in Ghana, Uganda and Brazil (Chapman and Mancini 2006). There is also UNFPA's Human Rights-Based Approach to Programming (UNFPA and Harvard School of Public Health 2010) which discusses their culturally sensitive, gender-responsive, human rights-based approach to programming; this deals particularly with UNFPA's three main areas of work: population and development, reproductive health and gender; it also covers humanitarian emergencies.

As a detailed example, this section considers the work of CARE International, who took up the challenge of incorporating a rights-based approach into all their work. This is of particular interest since their work was carried out all over the world, and they also subjected the approach they produced to evaluation. Material in this section draws on the information provided on CARE International UK's website (www.careinternational.org.uk) as well as the published report of the evaluation carried out (Picard 2005). Following this, other similar work will be discussed.

CARE International: a human rights-based organisation

CARE International is one of the world's largest independent relief and development organisations. It works in more than seventy countries and benefits over 45 million poor and marginalised people. It positions itself as a practical, hands-on organisation with thousands of programmes around the world that deal with the wide range of issues that keep people trapped in poverty, including HIV/AIDS, discrimination, lack of clean water, employment and/or living conditions, in other words, tackling the social determinants of health and working towards social justice. As they put it in their organisational mission: 'We seek a world of hope, tolerance and social justice, where poverty has been overcome and people live in dignity and security.' While CARE is a large international organisation, with more than 12,000 employees worldwide, they have strong local connections. They state that more than 90 per cent of staff are citizens of the countries where the programmes are run and who work with local contacts and expertise. CARE has no political or religious affiliation.

CARE aims to address the underlying causes of poverty, rather than to simply deal with its symptoms. CARE views poverty as the product of complex social processes that affect people's dignity and security as well as their material wellbeing and seeks to understand all the factors that make and keep people poor before choosing which ones to concentrate on in each individual project. They present as an example a mother in a rural African setting, who struggles to grow enough food for her family year after year. She could be struggling because drought or another natural disaster continually causes her crops to fail. But there may also be other reasons for her poverty. She might not have the skills to get the highest yield from her crops; she might be marginalised by people in her community, perhaps because she is HIV positive or is caring for a sick family member, and as a result faces a number of difficulties. To help decide how to tackle poverty they suggest that the causes of poverty need to be examined from three different perspectives: from the perspective of people's basic needs; from their position in society; and from the way the society in which they live works.

Projects then need to address each of these different perspectives. First, people's basic needs, for food, clean water and shelter, should be met, while also trying to assure that future generations can have these needs met as well. Second, work is needed to address dynamics in the social structure, to help all people to take control of their lives, and work towards ending inequity and discrimination. Third, work must focus on creating an enabling environment, including efforts to assure sound and equitable government, a supportive private sector and a thriving civil society. Addressing the underlying causes of poverty in this way helps improve the chances of developing sustainable solutions for the future.

In 2003, CARE moved to adopt an explicit human rights-based approach in their work, through the use of six programme principles: promote empowerment; work in partnership with others; ensure accountability and promote responsibility; address discrimination; promote the non-violent resolution of conflicts; and finally, seek sustainable results. They carried out a self-evaluation of the application of this rights-based approach in practice, examining sixteen projects from Bangladesh, Bolivia, Burundi, Cambodia, Guatemala, Honduras, India, Peru, Rwanda, Sierra Leone, Somalia and Thailand (Picard 2005). For each project they measured achievements against each of the six principles, as well as assessing local outcomes. Not all the projects were equally successful, but analysis of their different experiences offers some useful findings which can serve as guidance for future work. One key finding was that client groups and partners reported that more time and support were needed than for a conventional project. Obtaining the support of key stakeholders was not always possible at the outset, and required persistence, advocacy, transparency and negotiation. It was particularly important that any effort to raise awareness of rights and responsibilities relating to the problems facing marginalised groups include both rights-holders and duty-bearers, both of whom are equally capable of transformation. They also identified that attention needs to be paid to assessing, managing and taking risk, and this is relevant to staff and client groups alike. A rights-based approach needs variety and flexibility in use of participatory methods at all different stages, for needs analysis, problem diagnosis, option generation and appraisal, and finally for decision-making.

In terms of promoting empowerment, invariably, rights-based programming went beyond conventional levels of participation by beneficiaries and partners. Projects involved empowering marginalised groups to take control over their own lives as an integral part of understanding development and dignity as a basic human right. All projects took as their starting point the need to give voice to the most marginalised groups, whether or not the projects chose to invoke the language of rights. A few projects found that they needed to design quite elaborate processes to facilitate and mobilise community groups, while others demonstrated the importance of empowerment through solidarity.

By acting within a rights framework, CARE staff have found that they had to interact and work in partnership with a wide spectrum of players in order to build alliances to create a more powerful force for change and to forge links between rights-holders and duty-bearers. They also identify that it is particularly important to judge when to step back from leadership into a facilitator role, passing the lead to marginalised groups to let their voices be heard. They also note that engaging with a greater number of stakeholders means managing a complexity of relationships and this required skill and patience, and time.

While not all projects were directly aimed at improving CARE's accountability to the poor, the evaluation stressed that greater scrutiny of the relationship between CARE and poor communities is needed if RBAs are to be taken seriously. Furthermore, without proper engagement and research into social, cultural and economic differentiation, some social groups can be left out of a programme, mirroring their social exclusion. They conclude that exemplary relationships with marginalised people bear characteristics of trust, friendship and a 'journeying together'. One key finding in terms of promoting responsibility was that the process of dialogue between rights-holders and duty-bearers proved to be transforming for *both* groups. In most projects, this was accomplished by facilitating discussion and dialogue in an open and collaborative manner; while in others organised groups put pressure on responsible actors.

To oppose discrimination through its programmes, CARE has also looked internally at the views and attitudes of staff within the organisation. Dialogue amongst staff, partners and community members, for example, has in some cases created the energy and commitment to move forward towards elaborating a gender strategy. Projects did succeed in focusing attention on populations being discriminated against, and in recognising all forms of discrimination. Many examples addressed the double discrimination of women where norms and traditions subordinated women even within the most marginalised groups. Many projects found there was a direct link between opposing discrimination and opposing violence. Violence and rights abuses against marginalised or disenfranchised groups was a common theme, as many countries where CARE is working are recovering from war or affected by chronic conflict.

The evaluation report (Picard 2005) highlights that the poverty of specific groups of people is perpetuated by political or economic structures, social norms and even specific environmental conditions. By examining underlying causes of poverty, RBAs help to focus interventions on issues that may require a longer time horizon but can produce more sustainable results. In many of the projects featured, the root cause of the communities' poverty was linked to poor governance and/or social exclusion.

Having discussed the findings from looking at the six programme principles across all the projects, the work of one particular health-focused project is now examined, before summarising the conclusions from the evaluation in terms of a continuum of rights-based approaches. The Integrated Nutrition and Health Project was carried out in the state of Chhattisgarh in India. The project started in 2001, at which time the health situation was characterised by a high infant

Table 5.2 The Integrated Nutrition and Health Project: best practices

Aim	Best practice introduced
Communities should be able to demand and access services from the State	Strengthen local governance to take up health and nutrition issues as a priority during the quarterly Village Parliament
Enable people-centred advocacy on the Integrated Child Service Development Program	Introduction of Meet for Empowerment Learning & Advocacy (MELA) – a forum for learning and making needs heard to officials
Promote right to information on health	Social Audit conducted in several villages to make people more proactive about health and nutrition
Provide disadvantaged, malnourished children with better nutritional options	Revitalise the 'foster mother' (Dharam Dai) tradition to ensure essential nutrition

Source: derived from Picard (2005: 29)

mortality rate of 76 per 1,000 live births, and a high maternal mortality rate of 498 per 100,000 live births. The project reached 808,000 beneficiaries in the time up to 2004, and was based around the introduction, or reintroduction, of four 'best practices' (see Table 5.2). By disseminating these best practices, CARE sought to do a number of different things. First of all, it aimed to raise awareness among beneficiaries of the importance of nutrition and health interventions, and following this to bring about a change in those behaviours and practices within the rural community that accounted for high rates of infant and maternal mortality. It also sought to strengthen the health care system by building the capacities of government officials from the grassroots to the developmental block level to the district level.

All four innovations relied significantly on advocacy as a critical step. They also emphasised the voice and participation of women. The results from a project of this scale are multifarious. Communities, and especially women, began to voice their opinions and understand the problems. Responsible individuals and institutions became more accountable and transparent. Networks of officials and beneficiaries began to form, enabling the latter to voice their concerns and influence decisions. Information was shared more fully between villagers and service providers. Coverage and access to health and nutrition services improved as a result of the revitalisation of the Dharam Dai (foster mother), the incorporation of health and nutrition issues into local governance for the first time in the country and increasing pressure from grassroots women exercising their right to information. The project made best use of traditions and existing structures to create positive changes, not only in health and nutrition, but also in the general health of communities and their ability to raise their 'voice with dignity'.

Comparison across the projects evaluated suggested that it was appropriate to think in terms of a continuum of rights-based approaches (Figure 5.1), involving four identifiable stages. The first stage on this continuum is research, analysis and diagnosis, where use of a range of different participatory methods is important.

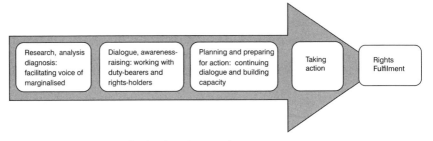

Figure 5.1 A continuum of rights-based approaches

The second stage is dialogue and awareness-raising, raising awareness of rights and responsibilities, fostering dialogues to achieve a common understanding of problems, creating safe space for discussion of sensitive or taboo subjects. The third stage comprises planning for action, proposing solutions and preparing the ground; here important components including building the capacity of duty-bearers for responsible action and facilitating the joint proposal or agreement of solutions. Finally, the fourth stage is that of taking action. Not all the projects included in CARE's evaluation progressed to the stage of taking action but the majority were able to increase knowledge of rights and responsibilities. Distinguishing individual interventions along this continuum so that it could be visualised how they might evolve proved a useful exercise. Although the continuum is divided into four stages, there is overlap between them and many of the individual projects consisted of a sequence of steps along it.

The analysis across the sixteen projects also identified the need for systematic examination of inequities. This extends to disaggregating within marginalised or excluded groups by gender and other relevant categories. This type of investigation is fundamental and relies for its validity on the participation of marginalised groups, and on a careful examination of the power relations existing in the community or communities concerned. Chapter 6 returns to the importance of this point in identifying where power relations in different situations can usefully be analysed as a part of a human rights analysis to evaluate the human rights implications of different policies and programmes.

The final point to draw from their analysis is about the use of human rights language and legislation. The examples spanned across a spectrum of rights: from moral rights (to be heard), and economic, social and cultural rights (to live in dignity and wellbeing), to legal rights (individual human rights or rights as a citizen). Not all projects perceived the need to invoke human rights legislation or frameworks. Explicit use was made by programmes that incorporated human rights into community education, or that were aimed specifically at achieving the legal rights of citizens. In other examples, rights language was minimised in favour of tapping into the values, beliefs and principles of the culture to achieve more equitable treatment of excluded groups.

In all the projects, evaluation identified promising signs of change: duty-bearers who responded to pressures or demands of marginalised groups; a greater ability in CARE to broach and discuss issues of inequity with clients and partners; whole communities that have taken control over decision-making processes; and myriad instances of marginalised groups no longer voiceless or faceless. A word of caution is in order. Perhaps it is still too early to tell if rights-based approaches do indeed achieve sustainable impact in the form of changing power relations in support of the excluded and marginalised. It was not always apparent from the individual projects how fully they grasped the complexity of power relations in their context; in some cases it appears that they did not probe those issues. A further question is whether, even with the evidence of change thus far, marginalised groups will, for instance, have the confidence and skills to continue to take risk, advocate or pressure others once CARE removes itself as the external facilitator.

Further documentation of CARE's RBA can be found in other projects and settings: work on the prevention of female genital cutting in Ethiopia and Kenya in East Africa reinforces these findings (Igras *et al.* 2004), as does work on the right to health in Peru (Frisancho and Goulden 2008), in collaboration with ForoSalud, a civil society network; and later work carried out by CARE USA and Oxfam America described by Rand and Watson (2008). Sarelin (2007) discusses a needs-based study carried out by CARE International in Malawi to establish the impact of HIV/AIDS on agricultural production and rural livelihoods, as well as to identify measures that could be taken to alleviate the situation. Her analysis highlights differences and similarities between needs-based and rights-based approaches, an essential difference being that rights-based analysis necessitates consideration of power, politics and struggles over resources.

Other rights-based approaches to programme design and planning

Increasingly, the literature is reflecting different applications of RBAs to programme design and planning. There is not space here for an exhaustive review; instead, a selection of the literature is discussed, focusing on those publications that have included some type of assessment or evaluation of the impacts of the use of the rights-based approach.

Berman (2008) reports on lessons learnt from documenting experiences and programmes that incorporated RBAs in several Asia-Pacific countries from 2004 to 2008, involving fourteen projects in countries as diverse as Bangladesh, India, Nepal, Cambodia, Indonesia, Laos, Vietnam, the Philippines and Fiji under the aegis of the Asia-Pacific UN Inter-Agency Lessons Learned Project (LLP) on the RBA to Development. WHO (2008b) brings together a range of different examples of a rights-based approach to the health components of poverty reduction strategies. Both of these demonstrate different success stories through the projects included, and to the limited extent that they offer conclusions across the different projects, they reinforce the findings from CARE International's evaluation discussed above.

Successful uses of rights-based approaches are also reported in a wide variety of projects working with different marginalised or disadvantaged groups. Perkins (2009) discusses the RBA used by a drop-in centre for vulnerable women in Cairo, including women who have low income, are displaced and /or refugees. The approach has helped women access basic health determinants. Paiva *et al.* (2010) document the success of a multicultural RBA in working on HIV prevention for young people with different religious communities (Catholic, Evangelical and Afro-Brazilian) in Brazil. Their analysis demonstrated success of the RBA in increasing inter-religious tolerance and building a common understanding of the sexuality and prevention needs of youth. Pillai *et al.* (2008) provide an example of successful rights-based HIV/AIDS work with people in prostitution and sex workers in rural India.

Mayhew *et al.* (2006) argue that NGOs need to be seen as duty-bearers who are required to uphold rights through their services, activities and principles of operation, in much the same way that CARE International discussed the responsibilities of their own staff and projects. Mayhew *et al.* discuss the difficulties this may cause in terms of funding policies that mitigate against adopting such a position. NGOs must ensure their three-way accountability: to government, to their clients and also to other civil society groups working in the area. They discuss their work in collaboration with NGOs delivering HIV-related services to prisoners and injecting drug users in Malawi and Pakistan and the framework for rights-based work for health that resulted, demonstrating how it helped the NGOs to develop their practice as well as monitoring their accountability.

There have also been examples of successful use of RBAs in European settings. In England, the Department of Health (2007) has identified five key aims of a human rights-based approach to health care: putting human rights principles and standards at the heart of policy and planning; empowering staff and patients with knowledge, skills and organisational leadership and commitment to achieve a human rights-based approach; enabling meaningful involvement and participation of all key stakeholders; ensuring clear accountability throughout the organisation; and finally, non-discrimination and attention to vulnerable groups. EHRC (2009a) presents the results of a major inquiry that examined progress towards the effectiveness and enjoyment of a culture of respect for human rights in Great Britain and considered how the current human rights framework might best be developed and used to realise the vision of a society built on fairness and respect, confident in all aspects of its diversity. The inquiry found a very clear reluctance on the part of many public authorities to use the specific language of human rights, but that where human rights language is used, for example in some police, health and education services, the effect is to enable staff and also to provide better protection for and application of human rights in service delivery. One part of the evidence provided to the inquiry (EHRC 2009b) presents the results of the experience of five different organisations, selected on the basis that they had a reputation for embedding human rights into their work: the Welsh Assembly Government, the National Policing Improvement Agency, Southwark Council, Mersey Care Trust and Age Concern (Cymru and England). While the report emphasises that work in each of these organisations is still in early stages, they identify that engagement with human rights has clear benefits for users, carers and communities as well as for staff and the organisations themselves. The report emphasises the importance of leadership, of human rights 'champions', training and engagement with communities and stakeholders (EHRC 2009b). Another part of the inquiry examined the role and experience of inspectorates, regulators and complaints-handling bodies in promoting human rights standards in public services through an interview-based study (EHRC 2009c); findings emphasised the importance of education, training and awareness-raising around human rights, and the particular importance of moving away from the dominance of legalistic language.

Turning to RBAs in health service provision, Simonelli and Fernandes Guerreiro (2010) report on an initiative of the International Network of Health Promoting Hospitals and Health Services to promote respect for children's rights in hospital, usually based around a charter for children's rights. From an application of their self-evaluation model in seventeen hospitals across nine countries in Europe plus Australia, they identify many aspects of good practice that demonstrate that respecting children's rights in hospital can result in a positive influence on both quality of service provision and health outcomes. However, they also identify a need for awareness-raising and training around rights in hospital staff, and report particular challenges in terms of lack of attention given to the right of children to information and participation.

The Scottish Human Rights Commission (the national human rights institution for Scotland) has published the results of its independent evaluation of a human rights-based approach used in the high-security forensic mental health institution for Scotland and Northern Ireland (SHRC 2009). The results provide practical lessons for other public authorities in the health and other sectors, as well as evidence of the value of adopting a human rights-based approach in three different areas. First, it led to improvements for staff as well as patients, namely a more constructive atmosphere with reduced staff stress, anxiety and fear. There was also a reduction in blanket policies and increased individual assessment of rights and risks and a more proportionate use of measures such as seclusion. The use of an RBA reduced risks, including organisational risks such as litigation. Finally, the RBA laid the foundation for integrating all other duties, including new equality, mental health and freedom of information laws. Among the key factors identified as responsible for success in adoption were: top-level buy-in and leadership; involving human rights expertise in all stages of audit and review; a participatory approach; and finally, the focus on everyone's rights, including those of staff.

Also within the UK context, a recent three-round Delphi consultation amongst experts in the field of domestic and sexual violence and abuse (Itzin et al. 2010a) concluded that a human rights framework was a required basis for policy and practice, with explicit attention to gender, sexuality, ethnicity, and disability within this. Itzin et al. (2010b) set out the details of what this framework would involve. Relatedly, Morgaine (2011), using the critique and experiences of women of colour, identifies the challenges within the mainstream domestic violence movement in the United States, and concludes that a human rights approach could address some of these concerns by supporting the necessary holistic approach to domestic violence and increasing coalition-building and community engagement.

Practice in individual care: rights-based approaches in individual interactions between health/welfare professionals and patients/clients

The use of rights-based approaches in the practice of individual health and welfare professionals is a topic that deserves a book in itself, however here it will be restricted to a short review only. Much of this work is discussed under other headings or labels. First of all, there is considerable overlap with various different codes of professional ethics. For example the 'Principles of the Ethical Practice of Public Health' of the American Public Health Association (Public Health Leadership Society 2002) start with a reference to the UDHR. Nixon and Forman (2008) explore complementary features of human rights and public health ethics, finding that each has something to offer to the other, and that they can thus act synergistically.

Curtice and Exworthy (2010) delineate a simple mnemonic encapsulating what they see as the human rights-based approach: human rights can be protected in clinical and organisational practice by adherence to the underlying core values of fairness, respect, equality, dignity and autonomy (FREDA). Their paper goes on to demonstrate that these principles are the basics of good clinical care as set out in current professional standards, such as the third edition of *Good Psychiatric Practice* (Royal College of Psychiatrists 2009), relating this to examples of clinical practice in the context of the UK's 1998 Human Rights Act and relevant decisions of the European Court of Human Rights. Asher *et al.* (2007), in a publication on 'the right to health' produced for the BMA and Commonwealth Medical Trust, include a section on a human rights-based approach to professional practice. In the field of reproductive and sexual health at the individual care level Cook *et al.* (2003) cover a wealth of examples. There can however be tensions between ethical and human rights standards, London (2008), discussing experience in South Africa, argues powerfully that unless the complementarities and differences in ethical and human rights standards, particularly acute in the problems of dual loyalty faced by clinicians, providers and policy-makers, are recognised, insufficient use of rights-based approaches will be made to impact the health of the most vulnerable in society.

Professional practice in disciplines such as occupational therapy, disability and social work is increasingly being focused around strengths-based and person-centred approaches that embrace shared decision-making (Pepin *et al.* 2010; Coulter and Collins 2011), and medical and other health professional practice increasingly focuses on patient-centred care, recognising its links to improved quality of life and reduced morbidity (Bauman *et al.* 2003). These approaches are highly correlated with rights-based approaches, although this link is not always explicitly made, and where it is, the discussion can often be in terms of 'patient rights' without making explicit connections to 'human rights'. See for example Groene (2011) and McClimans *et al.* (2011), who also discuss the links to clinical ethics. Ward and Moreton (2008) provide a very interesting discussion of a framework for addressing victimisation issues with sexual offenders, drawing on the resources of human rights theory and strengths-based treatment approaches. Birgden and Cucolo (2011), talking about the treatment of sex offenders more generally, argue that underpinning treatment approaches with human rights and professional ethics in a 'treatment as rehabilitation' approach is more effective than a 'treatment as management' approach; their arguments are very consistent with the findings of the evaluation of the human rights-based approach used in the high-security forensic mental health institution for Scotland and Northern Ireland (SHRC 2009) discussed earlier.

Within the disability field, professional practice has developed over the last twenty or so years in response to the demands to free practice from discrimination. The development of the International Classification of Functioning, Disability and Health or ICFDH (WHO 2001) has helped support this change. The ICFDH provides a common language for discussion of functioning, activity and participation in relation to a diverse spectrum of health conditions and can be applied to any individual; it avoids the need for the labelling of an individual as disabled or non-disabled, and recognises the importance of environment and social context in supporting or hindering participation in different activities. The ICFDH encourages attention to diversity.

The Centre for Human Rights (1994) and Ife (2008) consider how a human rights perspective can provide a unifying framework within which social work can be incorporated, while still accommodating cultural, national and political difference. Ife (2008) argues that a human rights perspective can strengthen social work, providing a strong base for practice that seeks to realise the social justice goals of social workers.

Empowerment education

> Where, after all, do universal human rights begin? In small places, close to home – so close and so small that they cannot be seen on any map of the world. Yet they are the world of the individual person: the neighborhood he lives in; the school or college he attends; the factory, farm or office where he works. Such are the places where every man, woman, and child seeks equal justice, equal opportunity, equal dignity without discrimination. Unless these rights have meaning there, they have little meaning anywhere. Without concerted citizen action to uphold them close to home, we shall look in vain for progress in the larger world.
>
> Eleanor Roosevelt at the presentation of 'IN YOUR HANDS: A Guide for Community Action for the Tenth Anniversary of the Universal Declaration of Human Rights', 27 March 1958, United Nations, New York, quoted from www.udhr.org

This final section on describing various types of rights-based approaches focuses on human rights education, referred to here as empowerment education, owing to the aim of such work to provide people with the tools to take control of their own lives and to participate in the different sectors of society. These approaches are concerned with making rights accessible to all, and concentrate on work with individuals or groups, often networked into and through different NGOs. The first section looks at a UK-based programme, called 'Active Learning for Active Citizenship'; although this was an explicitly rights-based approach, note that the title of the programme focused on active citizenship. Then a section on human rights education considers programmes that have been explicitly labelled as such, including the WHO cartoons on the right to health and HIV/AIDS.

Active Learning for Active Citizenship (ALAC)

Active Learning for Active Citizenship (ALAC) was a UK government-funded programme that took place over the period 2004–6, during which seven regional 'hubs' tried out a variety of approaches to citizenship learning for adults. The sources for the description in this section come from the various papers produced during the ALAC programme, accessed by the author in her role as one of the members of the steering group for the programme, two more formal reports on the structure of the programme (Woodward 2004) and the report by the external evaluators (Mayo and Rooke 2006), as well as the Take Part programme that followed ALAC, based on the national framework for active learning for active citizenship (Bedford *et al.* 2006) and its evaluation (Miller and Hatamian 2010). A book on the programme is also available (Annette and Mayo 2010), including chapters by the evaluators, from the facilitators, and from the different regional hubs, and the external evaluators have also written a paper (Mayo and Rooke 2008) which focuses on the participatory approach to evaluation that was adopted.

ALAC started by recognising and valuing local expertise, knowledge and experience and building upon these, emphasising the development of sustainable partnerships for the longer term. This was a community development-based approach, working towards empowerment, supporting organisations and groups within communities, and pursuing agendas for equity and social justice. Within the programme, there were seven different teams, each based in a different geographical location and each working with different constellations of groups and individuals. The seven teams formed the nucleus of seven regional hubs. The hubs organised into a network to learn from each other's experience, and an external team of evaluators was engaged.

Citizenship education was to start from local people's own perceptions of their issues and their learning priorities, negotiated in dialogue rather than imposed from outside. The hubs were intended as local people's provision – *their* provision, based in accessible premises, with a variety of programmes and activities tailored to local people's interests, driven by the priorities and aspirations of the learners themselves. Learner participation was to be central at every stage in the process: identifying learning priorities; developing the learning programme to be directly relevant to learners' interests and experiences; delivering the programme with the active involvement of the learners, with an emphasis upon the links between knowledge, critical understanding and active citizenship in practice; and subsequently evaluating the programme participatively.

Whilst the forms and levels of ALAC provision varied enormously across the hubs, there were a number of shared principles and approaches. Starting from people's own priorities and needs, ALAC emphasised experiential learning, processes of critical reflection and dialogue rooted in people's own experiences, both individually and collectively, through collective action. This drew upon the methods and approaches developed by the Brazilian educator Paulo Freire (1972) facilitating the development of critical consciousness and understanding, through cycles of action, reflection and then further action. In this model of learning, defined in terms of collective and critical reflection and dialogue, learners and learning providers learn together. To illustrate the diversity of the programme's activities the work of just three of the hubs is now outlined.

In the South West Region, the Speaking Up programme was run by Exeter Council for Voluntary Service for carers, people with mental health issues and people with learning difficulties. Learners gained the skills and confidence to speak up where it counts and to represent both their own and their interest group's issues. Through consultation with projects and working with co-tutors, the courses were continually developed. For example, a co-tutor recruited from the learning disability team in mid-Devon helped to develop active role play through her experience with a local drama group. Another co-tutor on a course for a mental health group was able to bring his own experiences, as a service user, to the design of the course.

West Midlands was the only ALAC hub targeting women specifically. At a time when gender issues had slipped down the policy agenda, the IMPACT programme, developed and delivered by the West Midlands hub, recognised the specific barriers and opportunities that women encounter when becoming active citizens. By working closely and flexibly with women, considering and addressing the practical barriers many women encounter, even when attempting to attend a course, the IMPACT programme built confidence and encouraged women to become questioning and challenging while developing self-awareness and a belief that they could make a difference. The West Midlands hub gradually and methodically engaged women and their families in effective community organising and increased their ability and confidence to exert influence at different levels of policy and service delivery.

In Lincolnshire, the initial focus of the hub's efforts was migrant workers, a group who are particularly hard to reach and particularly vulnerable as a result of language barriers, difficult and unpredictable working patterns, and a lack of information about their employment rights. The success of the Lincolnshire hub's work with migrant workers had at its core a flexible approach to promotion and outreach, for example, visiting temporary accommodation sites. In this context straightforward classroom-based, regular learning was unworkable due to the living and working conditions of the learners who were migrants working in agriculture. Learning provision was therefore extremely flexible, with an emphasis upon outreach work and one-off learning engagements and creative workshops, to cope with the problems associated with round-the-clock shift working. Learning provision and content was negotiated with migrant workers, and was based on identifying concerns that had sufficient relevance to ensure their engagement. The key issues and learning needs identified were around coping with their immediate living and working conditions: learning how to get a national insurance number and how to open a bank account, and learning about employment rights and housing law more generally. As well as supporting the improved citizenship experience of migrant workers in that process,

ALAC Lincolnshire has been actively working with groups of local service providers who are proactively taking their learning from the experiences and reflections of migrant workers into their organisations to improve services and joint working.

The ALAC evaluation demonstrated a wide range of positive outcomes. Participants in the programme gained increased confidence and skills in tackling local issues with service providers, and also reported positive change in health and wellbeing within their families. Individuals and groups became involved in service development and/or volunteering as trainers, became involved in formal volunteering and local networks, and also become more organised and involved in structured grassroots community activity. Participants learnt about and became more involved in governance structures. ALAC's wide range of outcomes included some that were planned and also a variety of multiplier effects of these, as active learning impacted not only upon individuals but also cascaded to impact upon their friends, families and communities. ALAC has led to beneficial ripple effects on services and service provision and the development of more effective forums and partnerships. In some of the evaluation workshops, participants mapped their influence at different levels: self, family, neighbourhood and community, local, regional, national and global.

In terms of change at the community level, some of the learning, and the impact of this learning within and between communities has taken place through facilitated workshops but at other times it has been the result of activities that have cascaded from ALAC. Communities have come together around common concerns, identifying their issues and training needs, sharing information between groups and communities, increasing dialogue between communities and raising community awareness about local services and how to access them. Groups and communities have been taking a more strategic approach in addressing the issues that affect them.

Participation in ALAC has enabled people to address the barriers that specific communities face. For example, intergenerational barriers were addressed through facilitating a dialogue around community safety issues across generational barriers (through an 'R u listening' programme). Many different health issues were also addressed, for example a local event for 500 women had stalls providing information on health issues such as domestic violence and breast cancer. Inter-cultural relations were enhanced by working together to find commonalities and connections, for instance through helping Muslim women to overcome language barriers and isolation, and working on children's involvement in activities in the month of Ramadan.

The participants' own words document examples of the impacts of the programme clearly, to give just four diverse examples:

> I have developed the drive to make change and the confidence to influence. At the same time I have been building up my knowledge of knowing where to influence.

> I went on to join (the local) Council. I became the rep for disabled people in the community and started getting involved in decisions affecting disabled

people in the community. I got involved with another rep and his organization – it has made a real difference and helped me to know someone else doing something similar and we have supported each other. Up until then I felt very isolated, I didn't know about these organizations and I realised there are a lot more people involved and doing things.

I'd lived there for 21 years – it had never dawned on me that we had nothing. There are 1500 properties and no services or amenities – not even a shop. This course definitely made me realise that wasn't right, that I could do something – it continually strengthened me.

I am Chair of the local Somali community organization. I have learnt a lot about government in London and I will be taking back that information to my community.

The evaluation of the ALAC programme produced findings with a considerable overlap with those from CARE's evaluation. First, they noted the time and support that this work takes. Secondly, the importance of involving key stakeholders was stressed. Thirdly, it required variety and flexibility in use of methods. Fourth is the need for careful attention to systematic analysis of inequities. Finally, tactical decisions were required as to the extent to use rights and rights language explicitly.

Over the two years of its life, the ALAC programme thus demonstrated promising signs of change; in particular, marginalised groups were becoming no longer voiceless or faceless. Questions remained about its sustainable impact however, as funding for continuation in the same form was not forthcoming. The work and its positive evaluation led to the production of a national framework for active learning for active citizenship (Bedford et al. 2006), and a further funded national programme, the Take Part programme, and network were created to continue the process of sharing resources and experience. Funding for Take Part was secured for 2009 to 2011, and there is also an associated programme of evaluation.

The interim evaluation (Miller and Hatamian 2010) indicates emerging trends, which will be investigated further in the final evaluation due in late 2011. First, the Take Part style of learning is most effective when developed in response to people's own issues and concerns, i.e. when the community development principle of starting where people are is followed. Learning is most successful when it is participatory and includes an element of critical reflection; there is a strong emphasis on increasing levels of civic participation through Take Part, which is seen as requiring long-term support structures. Where local government has a working relationship with the organisation or group facilitating Take Part, there is increased coordination of empowerment activities. Potential barriers and risks to the remainder of the programme include limited networking between organisations or groups at both regional and national levels. The varied and localised nature of the programme makes it difficult for external organisations to appreciate the Take Part offer; there is seen to be poor coordination between empowerment initiatives at a local level.

Human rights education

Turning now to human rights education that is explicitly labelled as such, first of all the two cartoon books produced by WHO are considered. These were both produced in the UN Decade on Human Rights Education (1995–2004), which argued that people need to be more aware of their rights so that they can take more control over their lives and that only then can effective action be generated to hold governments, and other powerful actors, accountable. The first of the cartoon books, on the right to health (WHO 2002b) aimed at making the right to health more widely known and understood as an instrument to empower those most in need, in recognition of the fact that improving awareness and understanding of the right to health is an essential prerequisite to operationalising this right. The second book, *HIV/AIDS Stand Up for Human Rights* (WHO 2003a, updated in 2010) was launched by the United Nations Office for the High Commissioner for Human Rights (OHCHR), the United Nations Joint Programme for HIV/AIDS (UNAIDS) and the World Health Organization (WHO). This second cartoon book was designed to empower young people to promote human rights in relation to HIV/AIDS, to raise awareness of the key linkages between HIV/AIDS and human rights, to demystify HIV/AIDS and to combat the myths and taboos associated with HIV and AIDS. Both cartoon books can be downloaded from WHO's website (www.who.int/hhr/activities/publications/en/index.html).

A growing amount of research demonstrates the value of human rights education. Kapoor (2007) demonstrates how human rights education played a significant role in addressing gender-caste discrimination in the state of Orissa in India, empowering the Dalit community, and Dalit women in particular, to take action. This has resulted in improvements at the very local level, in terms of initiatives such as better legal aid/support, and the establishment of police stations run by women, which will permit women to more easily report assaults against them, as well as advocacy for further change at state and national level. Kapoor (2007: 283) notes how human rights education, for the Dalit communities he discuss, changed 'their view of themselves and what is possible'.

Also in India, Bajaj (2012) in a study of school-based human rights education in Tamil Nadu illustrates the power of human rights education in government schools to bring about change in terms of pupils' agency and actions at school, home and in the community, while Kaushik *et al.* (2006) discuss activities at an institution of higher education for women, demonstrating the links between improvements in women's education, human rights and life chances.

Ramasubban (2008) examines the intersections between HIV/AIDS, sexuality and human rights in a paper on the history of resistance to the anti-sodomy law in India. This demonstrates how the struggle around a particular piece of legislation has acted to mobilise disparate alternative sexualities groups around a common strategy, thereby creating a loosely connected 'community' or prototype social movement. Ramasubban argues that going beyond legal reform in the direction of sexual rights, however, requires a broader coalition of groups, and a broad-based political agenda of sexual rights for all, which must critique patriarchy, dominant masculinity and sexual violence – forces that together govern both the subordination of women and repression of alternative sexualities.

Hopkins (2011) presents an interesting analysis of the difference between two contrasting approaches to human rights education: curriculum-based and experiential learning. The two programmes compared are both delivered by Amnesty International: a curriculum-based programme in Washington, DC, in the United States and experiential learning in Ouagadougou, Burkina Faso. She finds both methods were successful in empowering participants and increasing their impact as effective activists. She further argues that the effectiveness of these approaches can be enhanced by incorporating peer education approaches within both models.

Rights-based approaches: a growing industry

The examples discussed in this chapter demonstrate the positive effects that can result from the use of rights-based approaches. This does not mean that rights based-approaches represent some sort of 'magic bullet', a panacea for all ills. Additionally, as the examples of CARE International and ALAC illustrate, not all contexts or situations are suitable for advocacy that is *explicitly* based in human rights. A further example of this appears in the report of an inter-country meeting on health and human rights, organised by the WHO Regional Office for the Eastern Mediterranean (EMRO 2006). The meeting discussed the case of Palestinian women forced to give birth at Israeli checkpoints because they are not allowed to pass through to go to the nearest health facility. In this situation, they suggested that it is better to approach the situation from a health point of view rather than a human rights point of view.

A number of the examples discussed have highlighted the importance of power relations, calling for explicit attention to an examination of these as part of any rights-based approach. This remains an important area for further development as to different methods and tools that can assist in this process. One very helpful example to illustrate the possibilities is provided by Surjadjaja and Mayhew (2011). They present an analysis of policy change in relation to abortion over the period 2004 to 2006, using stakeholder analysis frameworks (Brugha and Varvasovsky 2000) to analyse the power, networking and political will of key actors, and how this influenced and was influenced by the framing of the issue as a health issue and/or a rights issue by the different stakeholder groups.

6 Evaluating the human rights effects of health and social policy

As noted earlier, health policies, programmes and practices can promote and protect *or* restrict and violate human rights. A single policy can promote some rights for some groups at the same time as violating the same rights for different groups or other rights for the same groups. This can be by design, neglect or ignorance. One important set of rights-based approaches are the various forms of human rights analysis that can be used to evaluate the human rights effects of health and social policy or programmes; some authors choose to talk about this in terms of a 'human rights impact assessment' analysis. There are an increasing number of these in existence and the future presents excellent prospects for further development in this field. Rather than examine them all in detail, this chapter focuses on elaborating just one of these approaches after a brief review of other approaches to human rights analysis. This example is one of the first approaches to appear in the literature, yet is surprisingly absent from later coverage in reviews such as Worm (2010); it also originated within a public health and human rights context, and is an approach that public health practitioners find accessible and useful, as judged by both the author's own students and those at Harvard and Johns Hopkins (Gostin and Laazarini 1997).

Human rights impact assessment as a separate framework began to be identified in the later 1990s (Bakker *et al.* 2009), and developed using the experiences of environmental, economic and social impact assessment. An assessment can be conducted prospectively, to predict the potential impact of interventions on the enjoyment of human rights, or retrospectively, to document the impact of interventions after implementation. Many of the assessment tools have a particular focus, so that the Health Rights of Women Assessment Instrument, HeRWAI, (Aim for Human Rights 2008), concentrates on the impact of policies on women's health rights, while the Right to Health Impact Assessment (Hunt and MacNaughton 2006; MacNaughton and Hunt 2009) examines potential impacts of policies, programmes and projects on the enjoyment of human rights, with a particular focus on the right to health. The People's Health Movement, building on the HeRWAI, has also produced a guide to the assessment of the right to health and health care at the country level (PHM 2006). WHO (2011) published a guide to assessing policy coherence in human rights and gender equality in health sector strategies; one example of its application is to the case of Yemen (Rostedt and Vogel 2009). Finally, a number of different policy analyses incorporate rights alongside other criteria: an excellent example is Lovvorn *et al.* (1997) who evaluate five alternative policies regarding HIV testing of pregnant women against five criteria: vertical and horizontal equity, avoidance of stigma, right to privacy, effectiveness and feasibility.

A seven-stage method of human rights analysis

In this chapter, the seven-stage approach, which is possibly the earliest specific human rights assessment tool to appear in the health literature, is discussed at some length. Originating in some of the early work on human rights and HIV/AIDS, a seven-stage approach to human rights impact assessment was outlined by Gostin and Mann (1994), and then elaborated in other publications including Gostin and Lazzarini (1997), and Gruskin and Tarantola (2001, 2005). The version presented here takes the basic seven stages as listed in the references by Gruskin and Tarantola, drawing on Gostin and Mann (1994) for their helpful coverage of the concepts of over- and under-inclusion and for some of the details in relation to the execution of the seven stages.

The tool has been applied to analyse a wide range of policies and programmes across the globe. Ford *et al.* (2010) present an analysis of when to start antiretroviral therapy in resource-limited settings. Bisaillon (2010) applies the method to examine the mandatory HIV screening policy for newcomers to Canada, and Chiswell, in Chapter 7, examines a peer education-based HIV/AIDS prevention programme for adolescents in South Africa (the GOLD programme). The applications of this form of human rights analysis are not just to HIV/AIDS however, and Chapters 8, 9 and 10 present examples in relation to specific policies or programmes for three other topics. At national level, Treacy in Chapter 10 examines the MindMatters programme implemented in secondary schools in Australia to promote mental health and wellbeing in students. At regional level, Singh in Chapter 8 analyses the mid-day meal scheme implemented in the Indian state of Madhya Pradesh, while Adamowitsch in Chapter 9 scrutinises the Styrian Tobacco Prevention Strategy in Austria.

Table 6.1 presents a summary of the seven-stage approach. At the outset, there are a few features worth noticing. First, although presented as a series of seven stages, it is not necessary to carry them out in order from stage 1 through to stage 7; the stages are interrelated, and answers to a stage later in the sequence may necessitate a return to parts of an earlier stage. Secondly, this form of human rights analysis can be carried out either prospectively, when a new policy/programme is being planned, or retrospectively to examine a policy or programme that has already been implemented.

Third, and perhaps most importantly, throughout the process of working through the different stages, it is necessary to think carefully about the power relations present in different societies and how these structure current patterns of discrimination, oppression and disadvantage within the communities and societies that the policy/ programme operates. As Chapter 2 emphasised, freedom from discrimination is a key right, and requires careful attention to ensure that benefits and risks are spread equally and do not reinforce existing patterns of disadvantage.

Table 6.1 The seven stage approach to human rights analysis

1. What is the specific intended purpose of the policy or programme?
    i. Who does it target?
    ii. Who does it exclude?
    iii. How does it work? What interventions/activities/mechanisms does it use?

2. What are the ways and the extent to which the interventions in the policy or programme may impact positively and negatively on health?
   For each intervention involved in the policy/programme:
    a. Is the form of intervention appropriate and accurate?
    b. Is the intervention likely to lead to *effective* action?
    c. Is there informed consent to participation?
    d. Is the intervention as cost effective as any alternatives?

3. What and whose rights are impacted positively and negatively by the policy or the programme?

4. Do the interventions in the policy/programme *necessitate* the restriction of human rights?

5. If an intervention does necessitate the restriction of rights, have the criteria/preconditions to restrict rights been met?

6. Are the health and other relevant structures and services capable of effectively implementing the policy or programme?

7. What system of monitoring, evaluation, accountability, and redress exists to ensure that that the policy or programme is progressing towards the intended effects, and that any adverse effects can be acted upon?

Source: elaborated from Gostin and Mann (1994); Gruskin and Tarantola (2005)

Stage 1: what is the specific intended purpose of the policy or programme?

At the outset of any analysis, a clear understanding of the purpose of the policy or programme is essential. It is to be hoped that any policy or programme description would be very clear on this matter, not least because this facilitates public understanding as well as facilitating monitoring and evaluation. Clarifying the specific purpose or purposes also offers an opportunity to expose prejudices, stereotypical attitudes and irrational fears. Accompanying a general statement of purpose, it is usual to find more specific aims, objectives and/or goals; the terminology used may vary considerably from place to place and time to time.

At this stage it is essential to recognise that the policy/programme of interest may have multiple purposes/components and, if this is so, these should be itemised separately. Identification of the population group(s) that the policy/programme is aimed at or targets may need to be done separately for each component. Alongside this, it is worth identifying what population groups are *not* covered by each component of the policy/programme.

The final element in the first stage is to identify the interventions, mechanisms and/or activities that the policy/programme contains, by which its purposes are to be achieved. Ideally the basic description of the policy or programme will set these out clearly in relation to specific goals in terms of health outcome, but sometimes a fair amount of work is necessary to identify these.

Stage 2: what are the ways and the extent to which the interventions in the policy or programme may impact positively and negatively on health?

This stage examines the evidence that exists for the effectiveness of the policy/programme, looking at what is known about documented positive health effects and negative health effects, examining both intended and, where there is evidence, unintended effects. At this stage the research evidence is brought to bear, and also, in areas where research evidence is lacking or even non-existent, expert opinion can be utilised. This may be vitally necessary where the analysis being carried out is of the use of some policy or programme in a distinctly different context or with a distinctly different population group to the contexts where any research evidence has been obtained. In carrying out this stage, the analysis needs to look in turn at each of the different interventions/mechanisms/activities by which the policy/programme is delivered.

In examining health effects, it is important to identify which population groups are affected in each case and explore whether the positive and negative effects occur in the same or in different population groups. Finally it can be helpful to distinguish between definite effects and possible effects, taking into account lack of certainty in the evidence base.

There are four subsidiary questions that can be used to guide the analysis of any particular policy, programme or component intervention: is the form of intervention appropriate and (where relevant) accurate?; does the intervention lead to action with the desired effects?; are there issues with informed consent?; and is the intervention as cost effective as any alternatives and what are the opportunity costs?

A useful example of how these questions can be applied is provided by considering the case of HIV screening, drawing here on the discussions in chapter 3 of Gostin and Lazzarini (1997). In applying the first question, 'is the form of intervention appropriate and accurate?' as part of considering the potential benefits and harms of screening, accuracy needs to be considered first. As Gostin and Lazzarini discuss, in HIV screening programmes, three sources of error exist. The first is testing during the 'window' period after infection but before antibodies are detectable. The second source of error comes from testing under adverse conditions, where there may be variations in the test kit, and there may also be human error. The third potential source of error is related to the prevalence of HIV infection in the target population for the screening programme. In low-prevalence situations, the positive predictive value (the proportion of patients with positive test results who are correctly diagnosed) is relatively low and there is a greater possibility of a false positive, something which is obviously undesirable. The net result of examining the first question in this case is obviously highly dependent on the particular context in which the screening programme is being considered or is being operated.

Now consider the second question, 'is the intervention likely to lead to effective action?' Here, in relation to HIV screening, what happens after positive status is detected needs to be considered carefully. It can be argued that the screening programme is valuable if it leads to valued outcomes such as prevention of HIV transmission *and/or* provision of health care (e.g. ARV) that is not otherwise accessible. This brings us into considering what happens after the screening itself or, equivalently, requires that there must be something more than just the screening itself.

Now to the third question: 'what about informed consent?' While both legal and ethical standards would suggest that public health programmes are based on informed consent, this is also an area where public health goals are sometimes held to require its omission. One example is the Unlinked Anonymous Prevalence Monitoring Programme in the UK (www.dh.gov.uk/ab/Archive/UASSG/DH_096938). This began in 1990 and aims to measure the distribution of infection, in particular HIV, in accessible groups of the adult population. The objectives of the programme include assessing the effectiveness of voluntary confidential testing for clinical diagnosis of HIV infection. Data obtained are also used in the production of estimates of numbers of HIV-positive people requiring treatment and care in the future, to help in the planning of services for those affected by HIV and AIDS and to help target and evaluate health promotion. A later stage in human rights analysis, stage 5, looks at whether the criteria or preconditions for justified restriction of rights are met by the policy/programme under scrutiny.

Finally, the fourth question considers 'is the policy/programme as cost effective as any alternatives? And what are the opportunity costs?' This is perhaps the question that is most difficult, if not impossible, to answer, or at least to answer fully, since the current evidence base is not sufficient in many cases. The concept of opportunity cost may be useful, this can be understood as examining the cost of something in terms of an opportunity forgone (and the benefits that could be received from that opportunity), or alternatively as the most valuable forgone alternative.

To continue with the HIV screening example, here it would be important to consider the purpose of the HIV screening programme, alongside possible alternative purposes. There may be different alternatives to be considered if the purpose is behaviour change/transmission reduction than if it is access to treatment. Note also that opportunity costs may rise sharply if informed consent is not present (Gostin and Mann 1994). Certain populations (e.g. commercial sex workers or people with multiple sex partners or migrants) are often targeted for mandatory screening, yet this may alienate these communities and fuel the behaviours that the policies seek to prevent. This illustrates how particular aspects of the way a policy/programme is implemented may affect the likelihood of effective action resulting; alternatives such as empowerment of individuals to negotiate safer sex and/or improvement of women and children's economic and social situation might well be more cost-effective in this example.

Stage 3: what and whose rights are impacted positively and negatively by the policy or programme?

The third stage in the human rights analysis examines the human rights implications of the policy or programme. Many policies and programmes affect autonomy, privacy or equity in some way; the question that needs to be explored in each of these areas is whether the benefits accruing outweigh limitations and whether there is any discrimination at work. This includes examining whether the policy or programme is discriminatory in some way that cannot be justified.

Evaluating the human rights effects of health and social policy 107

Policy aim: Protection from SARS (Severe Acute Respiratory Syndrome)

Intervention: Quarantine of all entrants from overseas

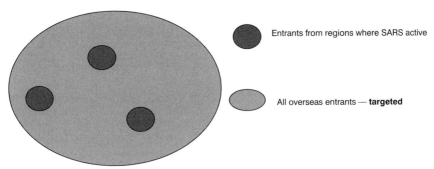

Figure 6.1 Over-inclusion: an example

Policy aim: Prevention of tuberculosis

Intervention: DOTS – Directly Observed Treatment Short-Course

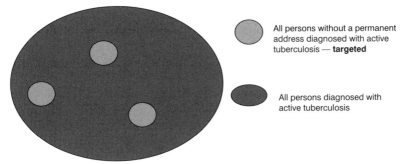

Figure 6.2 Under-inclusion: an example

One important question for examination in this stage is whether the policy or programme is well-targeted. This can be divided into examination of three distinct questions. First, it should be examined whether there is any over-inclusion, where the policy/programme is delivered to more people than necessary in order to achieve its objective. Second, it should be examined whether there is any under-inclusion, where the policy/programme reaches some, but not all, of the people it needs to reach in order to achieve its objective. The third question for examination is then: is there an alternative policy which is more humane, less restrictive, coercive or punitive? For each of these questions, the research evidence and/or expert opinion about alternatives needs to be consulted.

The concepts of over- and under-inclusion deserve some explanation. Figures 6.1 and 6.2 illustrate these concepts. In Figure 6.1, the policy aim of protection from Severe Acute Respiratory Syndrome (SARS) is considered, and as a possible intervention quarantine of *all* entrants from overseas. The target for the intervention in the figure is represented by the large lightly shaded oval, and it can be seen that this covers a much larger group that those that actually pose the risk, namely entrants into the country from regions where SARS is active. The intervention is thus over-inclusive. Over-inclusion does not necessarily violate human rights; in this case it does through affecting rights to freedom of movement. Even if rights are not affected, over-inclusion may well not be cost-effective. The question of whether rights are necessarily affected by the intervention, and if so, whether this is justified or not is considered in the next two stages of the analysis.

Figure 6.2 considers an example with a policy aim of prevention of tuberculosis, where the intervention considered is the use of Directly Observed Treatment Short-Course (DOTS). If the intervention is targeted only at people without a permanent address diagnosed with active tuberculosis (the small lightly shaded circles), this is only a subset of all persons diagnosed with active tuberculosis (the darker shaded oval). This targeting of the intervention is thus under-inclusive. By itself, under-inclusion does not necessarily pose a human rights problem, it may reflect an incremental approach to tackling the issue, reflecting a country's health or public health priorities within a situation of resource constraint. On the other hand under-inclusion may mask discrimination.

It is important to recognise that interventions contained within policies or programmes can be both over- *and* under-inclusive. For example, following Gostin and Mann (1994), consider a policy that aims to reduce transmission of sexually transmissible infections (STIs) through penalties against sex workers, but not their agents or clients. This is over-inclusive because there are some sex workers: who are not infected with any STI; who inform clients of potential risks; and/or who practise safer sex. At the same time it is under-inclusive because: it selectively targets a vulnerable population when the risky behaviour would not occur without the participation of others (clients and possibly also agents); it excludes all others (those who are not sex workers) who have sex without disclosing their infection status to partners.

It is at this stage that it is helpful to draw on some sort of analysis of power or prestige relations in the society or community in which the policy or programme is being or is to be implemented in order to explore whether the rights to participation and information of the least powerful groups are as respected as those of more powerful or prestigious groups.

Stage 4: does the intervention in policy or programme necessitate the restriction of human rights?

Within the fourth stage of the analysis, the different interventions or activities are scrutinised for whether they necessitate the restriction of human rights or not. This involves consideration both of the particular rights involved, and the particular groups affected, given the targeting of the policy/programme. It is important to consider both how the rights of those targeted are affected, and whether the rights of those *not* targeted are affected by virtue of being omitted. It is helpful to consider different subgroups within the population and how/if they are affected differently, so it is useful to think about: age, gender, sexuality, socio-economic status, ethnicity, culture, religion, language, place of residence, disability, acute/chronic health condition, etc. This is a second point at which power relations can usefully be considered, to examine whether the rights of the powerful are protected at the expense of the less powerful.

In terms of identifying which rights are affected, obviously those contained in the UDHR are relevant in all UN member states, and then there are also the rights contained in the group of treaties and conventions ratified by the country concerned. It is also necessary to consider any relevant regional documents, relevant national documents and relevant local documents, for example at state level in a federal country.

The most frequently relevant rights are the rights to freedom of movement, privacy and information, and freedom from discrimination, although other rights may be affected by particular policies/programmes and this possibility should be considered. So, the analysis needs to examine whether there are elements of the programme/policy that are coercive, restrictive or punitive; for example, is there any compulsory admission or detention, compulsory medication/treatment and/or compulsory participation? In terms of the right to freedom from discrimination, this is where consideration of programme/policy targeting is particularly important as the inclusion or exclusion of particular groups may amount to discrimination. Where the policy/programme involves the provision of some service, it is also important to consider accessibility, acceptability and quality, along the different dimensions set out in elaborations of the right to health in General Comment 14, discussed in Chapter 2 and summarised in Table 2.4.

Stage 5: if an intervention does necessitate the restriction of rights, have the criteria/preconditions to restrict rights been met?

Where stage 4 has identified that rights are restricted or compromised by some intervention in the policy or programme, then stage 5 in the analysis examines whether these restrictions can be justified or not. This requires a number of different steps. The first step is to review the circumstances in which rights can be restricted or limited, as discussed in Chapter 2, and consider whether these apply in the case of the policy/programme under consideration or not. As Chapter 2 discussed, there are situations where it is considered legitimate to restrict rights in order to achieve a broader public good, such as public health. The Siracusa principles (see Table 6.2) provide guidance to help assess whether any rights limitations are valid or justified. Table 6.2 also shows the criteria formulated for use where restriction of rights is being argued for on the grounds of protection of the public health.

In applying the Siracusa principles, a number of aspects need to be stressed. First, it is important to note that the law referred to in criterion 1 is the law of the country concerned. It should also be noted that there are value judgements involved in assessing whether the objective is legitimate and of general interest (criterion 2), and agreement on this may not be widespread in any society. Criterion 3 refers to 'strict' necessity, and while this seems relatively straightforward, limitations in the public health evidence base can make this difficult to determine.

Table 6.2 The Siracusa principles and criteria for justification of restriction of rights on grounds of protection of public health

Siracusa principles	Public health criteria
When a government limits the exercise or enjoyment of a right, this action must be taken as a last resort and will only be considered legitimate if the following criteria are met: 1. the restriction is provided for and carried out in accordance with the law; 2. the restriction is in the interest of a legitimate objective of general interest; 3. the restriction is strictly necessary in a democratic society to achieve this objective; 4. there are no less intrusive and restrictive means available to reach the same goal, and; 5. the restriction is not imposed arbitrarily, i.e. in an unreasonable or otherwise discriminatory manner.	In the case of restriction on the grounds of protection of public health, the following specific criteria should be met: 1. risk posed should be demonstrable and significant; 2. proposed interventions should be demonstrably effective; 3. approach should be cost-effective; 4. sanctions should be least restrictive necessary; 5. policy should be fair and non-discriminatory.

Source: ECOSOC (1984), Gostin (quoted in Coker (2001)), Gostin and Mann (1994)

For the first point of the public health criteria, note the explicit statement that the risk must be *significant*. Gostin and Lazzarini (1997: 66) explain this well:

> Significant risk must be determined on a case by case basis through fact specific individual inquiries. Blanket rules or generalizations about a class of persons with HIV infection do not suffice. The risk must be 'significant', not merely speculative or remote. For example, theoretically, a person could transmit HIV by biting, spitting, or splattering blood, but the actual risk is extremely low (approaching zero). Likewise, an HIV-positive [substitution for infected] health professional who does not perform deeply invasive procedures is highly unlikely to transmit HIV to a patient. Present knowledge does not support screening or excluding that person from the health care profession because, lacking a real and substantial possibility of HIV transmission, such policies do not meet the significant risk test.

Where there are any breaches of the Siracusa principles or the public health criteria, it should be noted carefully which criteria are concerned, and most particularly for which population subgroup(s) this applies.

Stage 6: are health and other relevant structures and services capable of effectively implementing the policy or programme?

The sixth stage switches the focus to possible issues connected with the implementation of the policy or programme. The first task is to identify whether there any factors which might interfere with implementation. For any such factors identified, it is then important to explore whether they apply equally in all situations (places, different groups in the population). This allows for determination of whether these factors may effectively discriminate against particular groups in the population.

This stage is also the place for careful consideration of the evidence of the effectiveness of the interventions that make up the policy or programme. Was that evidence gathered in similar settings to that in which the policy or programme is to be implemented? If not, will the differences in setting affect the likelihood of successful implementation? Here findings from implementation research into the particular intervention(s) can be examined to see what is known about barriers or facilitating factors for successful implementation and an assessment made about whether these operate or are likely to come into play in the setting under consideration.

Stage 7: what system of monitoring, evaluation, accountability and redress exists?

The final stage in the analysis focuses on the areas of monitoring, evaluation, accountability and redress. This explores the existence (or not) of monitoring and evaluation systems, trying to identify who is responsible for each of these, what happens to the reports produced and how freely available these are, to interested individuals and to different stakeholder groups. It is also important to examine what kind of information is routinely provided and to whom.

A second important area is that of the system or systems for complaints and feedback. First, it is important to examine whether these even exist. If they do, are they well-publicised and easy to access? Are they equally accessible to all different population groups and is assistance available to different groups who might have difficulty raising any complaint/feedback, and to the least powerful groups in society? For any system that does exist, it is important to assess its relationship to the policy/programme provider. For example, is it independent of the policy/programme provider?

Human rights analysis in practice

Using a range of examples from around the globe, the use of human rights analysis is illustrated by four examples presented in Chapters 7 to 10 below, drawn from analyses carried out in the last five years by public health practitioners. The choices made illustrate a range of different topics, as well as application at international, national and subnational level. The four different analyses also bring out some different general points about health and human rights analysis. In Chapter 7, Chiswell examines the peer education-based HIV/AIDS prevention programme for adolescents in South Africa (the GOLD programme). Her analysis illustrates the tension between reducing discrimination and trying to ensure effective implementation. The GOLD programme is limited to organisations who can fulfil a range of capacity criteria and who are already working with the target group. As Chiswell points out, there may well be areas with high prevalence and incidence of HIV/AIDS but which are not serviced by any organisation interested or able to implement such a programme.

At regional level, Singh in Chapter 8 analyses the mid-day meal scheme implemented in the Indian state of Madhya Pradesh. He draws attention to features of the implementation within Madhya Pradesh that widen the positive human rights effects of the programme, through the provision for appointing cooks from scheduled castes and scheduled tribes, thereby providing important employment opportunities to disadvantaged groups. He also draws attention to the monitoring of gender equity. Adamowitsch in Chapter 9 also presents a regional analysis, as she scrutinises a subset of the aims of the Tobacco Prevention Strategy in the state of Styria in Austria. She identifies potential discrimination in the strategy's effects: some interventions are only accessible to those with adequate levels of spoken German, although the state has a significant minority (9 per cent) of migrants. The aims she scrutinises do not involve any question of restriction of rights, being based on voluntary participation. Finally, at national level, Treacy in Chapter 10 examines the MindMatters programme implemented in secondary schools in Australia to promote mental health and wellbeing in students. She identifies a number of areas where discrimination is evident, affecting early school leavers, rural and remote students and, potentially, students with mental health problems. She also identifies concerns regarding language-appropriateness of the project for students from non-Western societies.

Reading across these selected points from the analyses described in Chapters 7 to 10 reinforces the importance of examining the actual and potential discriminatory effects of particular policies and interventions, and the difficulties of achieving a policy that does not discriminate. All four analyses also serve to illustrate the interrelated nature of many rights and how careful design of policies offers opportunities to promote and fulfil rights connected to the social determinants of health as well as working directly on health.

7 Addressing the sexual and reproductive health needs of adolescents in South Africa

A human rights analysis of the GOLD peer education programme

Melika Chiswell

Adolescents make up a fifth of the world's population, are the parents and workers of the next generation and yet only relatively recently has it been recognised by the global health sector that they have distinct and separate health care needs from those of adults, particularly in the area of sexual and reproductive health (Mngadi *et al.* 2008). Such inattention to their specific health needs leads to a range of negative outcomes, such as unwanted pregnancies, acquisition of sexually transmitted infections, including HIV/AIDS, and sexual violence. This is borne out by the reality that, worldwide, young people under the age of 25 experience the greatest burden of sexually transmitted infections (STIs) and the main cause of death amongst female adolescents is from unsafe abortions (Mngadi *et al.* 2008). The experience of poor sexual and reproductive health during adolescence can be long-lasting and often continues to impact young people's lives well into their adulthood (Bayley 2003; Bearinger *et al.* 2007; Rani and Lule 2004).

It was only in 1994, at the International Conference on Population and Development (ICPD), that adolescents were first defined as a significant and distinct group. It was acknowledged that they need specialised consideration and service provision in any global or local attempt 'to improve sexual and reproductive health, foster reproductive rights and stabilise the world's population' (Glasier *et al.* 2006: 1565).

At the same ICPD conference, sexual and reproductive health was defined, also for the first time, as a human right. It was stated that it is the

> right of men and women to be informed and to have access to safe, effective, affordable and acceptable methods of family planning of their choice, as well as other methods of their choice for regulation of fertility which are not against the law, and the right of access to appropriate health-care services that will enable women to go safely through pregnancy and childbirth and provide couples with the best chance of having a healthy infant.
>
> (UNFPA 1994: para 7.2)

In South Africa, where between 4.9 and 5.7 million people are living with HIV/AIDS (the highest burden in the world) a quarter of those affected are under the age of 15 years (Barron and Roma-Reardon 2008). Ninety per cent of all new HIV infections are in women, between the ages of 15 and 24 (Pettifor et al. 2005; Simbayi et al. 2005). Amongst sexually experienced adolescents, 2 per cent of males and 10 per cent of females report having been forced into sex. Twenty-eight per cent of females say their first sexual experience was unwanted (RHRU 2003).

In an attempt to address the overwhelming and very real sexual and reproductive health needs of South Africa's adolescent population, particularly in the area of HIV prevention, numerous programmes and campaigns have been initiated, with varying success, across the country. The GOLD Peer Education Development Agency is a peer education programme developed and run within South Africa. Considered to be very successful in its curriculum and approach, the programme has now been implemented in several other African countries. Using the human rights analysis tool proposed by Gostin and Mann (1994) and discussed in Chapter 6, the following is an assessment of the GOLD programme with regard to its impact on the human rights of the adolescents taking part.

Intended public health purpose of the GOLD programme

The GOLD (Generation Of Leaders Discovered) Peer Education Development Agency is a non-profit organisation established in South Africa in 2004 'to respond pro-actively to the increasing incidence of HIV infections amongst youth' (GOLD n.d.). GOLD's mission is to provide support to community organisations throughout sub-Saharan Africa in the 'sustainable roll-out of quality, youth, peer education programmes, in alignment with the GOLD model, thereby empowering youth peer leaders to become positive role models and agents of community change' (GOLD 2007: 1). The programme is currently being implemented in South Africa, Botswana and Namibia. Within South Africa and Botswana there are thirty-six community organisations implementing the programme in 122 secondary schools and associated communities, 208 trained and active programme facilitators and more than 7,400 school-aged peer educators (GOLD n.d.). The programme's strategic goals are:

1 To decrease the rate of new HIV infections amongst young people by promoting safe and healthy behaviours amongst those already infected with HIV and those not.
2 To alleviate the impact HIV/AIDS has on young people, orphans, children, their families and local communities.
3 To develop the capacity and leadership of community organisations already working with young people from communities with high rates of risk-taking behaviour amongst its young people; a high prevalence rate of HIV/AIDS; and large numbers of children who are orphaned and/or vulnerable.

(GOLD 2007)

In order to achieve these strategic goals the programme's target group is adults and youth leaders from community organisations whose own target group is young people from communities with high incidence and prevalence rates of HIV, large numbers of orphans, a lack of positive adult role models and high risk-taking behaviour amongst the young people (GOLD n.d.). The intended beneficiaries of the GOLD programme are the young people trained to become peer educators, the peers they then interact with and their surrounding communities.

Participating community organisations nominate facilitators within their organisation to recruit, train and support the peer educators throughout the programme, which lasts for three to four years. Topics covered during the training sessions include: self-development, sexual and reproductive health including HIV/AIDS, group work, presentation, facilitation and communication skills, leadership, advocacy and child rights, community development, mentoring, project management and research (GOLD n.d.).

The developers of the GOLD model believe that the programme addresses the root issues of HIV/AIDS in sub-Saharan Africa and it aims to achieve twenty-two developmental outcomes, which include an increase in: knowledge of HIV/AIDS; life skills; service access; healthy relationships; youth-led community activities; condom use; reports of delayed sexual debut; perceived efficacy of contraception use; and increased testing for sexually transmissible infections, including HIV. A decrease is expected to occur in relation to the experience of: sexual coercion; gender violence; substance abuse; school truancy; teenage pregnancy; the number of sexual partners in those sexually active; and fewer behavioural and disciplinary problems.

South Africa has between 4.9 and 5.7 million people living with the HIV infection, a quarter of whom are under the age of 15 years (Barron and Roma-Reardon 2008). Young women between 15 and 24 are at particular risk as they experience 90 per cent of all new HIV infections (Simbayi *et al.* 2005; Pettifor *et al.* 2005). The major factors believed to contribute to such a high HIV infection rate in South Africa are: high-risk heterosexual behaviour (unprotected sex, multiple partners and ignorance of HIV status); population mobility; substance use; high rates of sexually transmitted infections; elevated viral loads from recent infection or advanced disease; and significant vulnerability as a result of poor socio-economic conditions (Barron and Roma-Reardon 2008). Despite the largest roll-out programme globally of antiretrovirals South Africa has made little progress in slowing or reducing the spread of HIV (London 2002). In light of this almost totally overwhelming situation in regard to HIV/AIDS, programmes, policies and national initiatives are desperately needed to address this health issue, particularly the sexual and reproductive health needs of the country's young people.

Evaluation of the GOLD programme's likely effect

An impact study carried out by GOLD in 2008 (GOLD 2008a), in respect of the programme's anticipated developmental outcomes, found that programme facilitators, peer educators and their peers believed the programme had been most effective in: reducing substance abuse amongst the young people; decreasing the rate of teenage pregnancies; increasing the number of those involved in school or community leadership positions; improving behaviour in school and increasing knowledge of HIV/AIDS (GOLD 2008a). However, they also felt that there was least impact on: increasing contraception and condom use; testing for sexually transmissible infections (STIs); and reducing the number of sexual partners. This is somewhat concerning as these are the particular behaviour outcomes that prevent the spread of HIV, STIs and unintended pregnancies. According to the GOLD programme developers, gaining a true picture of the programme's impact on these more personal areas is very difficult as many young people state that they do not feel comfortable answering such questions.

Peer education involves educating and training a group of young people about a certain issue, such as sexual health and HIV/AIDS, who then impart their newly acquired knowledge and information to their peers (White et al. 2009). The aim is to increase general knowledge of certain issues and ultimately cause behaviour changes that will lead to better health outcomes. The underlying assumption of this approach is that 'people are most likely to change their behaviour if liked and trusted peers are seen to be changing theirs' (Campbell et al. 2005: 472). The support and evidence for this approach and its level of effectiveness appears to be quite mixed amongst the published literature. According to the Department of Human Services (2000), Aggleton (1997), White et al. (2009) and Kim and Free (2008), peer-led sexual health education programmes can be an effective way of imparting knowledge to young people about issues such as HIV/AIDS and condom use. However, whether or not the attainment of such knowledge actually leads to behaviour change and positive health outcomes, such as an increase in condom use and a decrease in newly acquired sexually transmitted infections, is not so clear. Sustained behaviour change is also difficult to be sure of. According to James et al. (2006), despite there having been many peer- or teacher-led sexual health programmes developed and run in South Africa, there is a significant lack of published evaluations of these programmes to show their level of effect. Kim and Free (2008) add that there is some evidence to suggest that such programmes benefit the peer educator to a much greater degree than the peers they are educating, in terms of development of self-esteem, self-efficacy, health knowledge and confidence.

Nevertheless, there does remain fairly strong support for a peer education approach, as long as several key issues are considered or included. Both the Department of Human Services (2000) and Aggleton (1997) argue that the most effective peer-led sexual health education programmes are those that are well planned, have clear objectives, adequate training, support and supervision and are regularly evaluated and monitored. The Department of Human Services (2000) add that programmes implemented over a sustained period of time and which seek to achieve behavioural outcomes are the most effective in sustaining behaviour change.

Internal monitoring and evaluation of the GOLD programme is incorporated into the curriculum, giving programme presenters ongoing feedback as to the programme's impact on participants. Many of the expected developmental outcomes are behavioural, such as an increased use of contraception and HIV testing. Peer educators receive intensive training for three to four years, much longer than any similar programme presented in the published literature and participating organisations are expected to continue the programme after GOLD withdraws its involvement.

A formal, well-designed and more objective evaluation of this programme, with regard to its sustained presence and long-term effects would be greatly beneficial in demonstrating its effect and value.

Appropriateness of the GOLD programme's target group

Young people are one of the most vulnerable groups at risk of HIV infection in South Africa. According to Hendricksen *et al.* (2007), a nationally representative household survey carried out in 2003 found that more than 15 per cent of young women and almost 5 per cent of young men, between the ages of 15 and 24 years old, were HIV positive. This is a population group in desperate need of attention and effective health initiatives if the country's HIV epidemic is to be addressed at all. There have been many previous HIV prevention programmes, conducted through the media, schools and communities, but which so far appear to have proved largely unsuccessful in reducing the incidence of HIV infection amongst the adolescent population (Agha 2002; Campbell *et al.* 2005).

In order to be eligible to run the GOLD programme an organisation has to show that they are already working with adolescents (including early school leavers) and are based within a community that has a high incidence and prevalence of HIV, a high number of orphans and vulnerable children, a lack of adult role models and a high number of young people demonstrating at-risk behaviour. Such programme inclusion criteria attempt to ensure that the most vulnerable and at-risk young people benefit from what it has to offer.

One area for consideration is that it appears from the literature provided by GOLD that the responsibility for addressing the sexual and reproductive health needs of young people is placed primarily on the shoulders of the young people involved in, and the recipients of, the programme. This seems to overlook the fact that people's behaviour and choices are influenced by more than just their peers but also the social context within which they find themselves, such as family and cultural expectations, socio-economic status, future aspirations and experiences of crime and violence. According to Campbell *et al.* (2005) HIV prevention initiatives need to incorporate or work closely with social development programmes so as to 'promote young people's social and political participation, increase opportunities for their economic empowerment, challenge negative social representations of youth, and fight for greater recognition of their sexuality and their right to protect their health' (Campbell *et al.* 2005: 471). The GOLD programme does advocate a community development approach but intends to achieve this through the actions of young people becoming more involved in their community.

Another aspect to consider regarding the programme's target group is that it is not made obvious from the promotional literature provided by GOLD (GOLD n.d.) whether the programme is inclusive of young people who engage in same-sex sexual relationships. Although HIV transmission in South Africa is primarily through heterosexual intercourse, same-sex-attracted young people are still at risk of HIV/ AIDS. If heterosexual-centric language is used in the programme, this may exclude a group of adolescents who are still at risk of HIV infection (Aggleton 1997).

Possible human rights burdens

The right to health, a fundamental human right, is 'dependent on, and contributes to, the realisation of many other human rights' (WHO 2008a: 6). Restrictions on or violations of human rights can have profound impacts on health outcomes both at the individual and population level (Jürgens and Cohen 2007). The GOLD peer education programme does not appear to cause any direct restriction of human rights. Organisations which implement the GOLD programme do so voluntarily and peer educators are recruited through a voluntary process and can cease to be involved at any stage with no sanction (GOLD n.d.). The GOLD model claims to have used a values- and rights-based approach in the development of its curriculum and the training and support provided to peer educators (GOLD n.d.). However, no further elaboration is given to demonstrate this claim.

As touched on earlier, the sole focus of the GOLD peer education programme is to enable young people to begin to address and impact the rates of HIV/AIDS amongst the adolescent population. Although this is a vital and important intervention, it does seem that this population group have been burdened with the sole responsibility of addressing this health issue, which in fact affects and is the responsibility of the county's entire population, its government, policy-makers, funding bodies and service providers. Of course it is acknowledged that such an organisation may not have the funds or special knowledge to work in other areas and, according to the Department of Human Services (2000), health promotion initiatives that spread themselves too thinly by trying to do 'everything' are much less effective than those that focus on a particular area of need. However, if the GOLD programme were to develop partnerships or align themselves with other organisations who work to lobby the public and private sectors, the media and service providers, this might help to ensure that the range of sexual health needs of adolescents, such as adequate service provision, are adequately addressed at a national level by the range of relevant stakeholders (CRC 2000).

Possible less restrictive alternatives that can achieve the same public health objective

According to the International Covenant on Cultural and Political Rights (ICCPR), it is acceptable to consider the restriction of human rights when it is in the interests of the greater good (Gostin and Mann 1994). If such restriction is necessary this should only occur after the criteria of the Siracusa principles (ECOSOC 1984) have been met. As Gostin and Mann (1994) point out, public health policies and programmes that do not involve coercion are considered to be the least restrictive on people's human rights. The GOLD peer education programme does not use any form of coercion to recruit implementing organisations or peer educators, nor does the programme restrict their human rights, in terms of freedom of speech, movement and thought, nor does it discriminate in terms of sex, religion or race (GOLD n.d.). In fact by providing young South Africans with greater knowledge, skills and confidence regarding their own sexual and reproductive health, they are being enabled to experience greater freedom of their rights to choice, self-determination and health-impacting decisions, which they may otherwise have been denied without such knowledge and support (WHO 2008a).

Are relevant structures and services capable of effectively implementing the GOLD programme?

In order for organisations to be eligible to implement the GOLD peer education programme they have to demonstrate adequate infrastructure to support the programme in both the short and long term (GOLD n.d.). They need to address eleven capacity criteria, which include: an effective organisational management structure; a history of resource mobilisation and the ability to raise sufficient funds for running costs; active engagement of relevant community stakeholders, for example police and health clinics; and a proven ability to manage and account for funds used (GOLD n.d.). The same selection criteria are applied to all organisations that apply to implement the GOLD peer education programme. Based on the information provided, along with consideration of GOLD's regional and site selection criteria, which relates to where the need is greatest, i.e. the highest incidence and prevalence of HIV, high numbers of orphans and vulnerable children, poor adult role models and significant youth risk behaviour, a decision is made as to whether or not the GOLD programme will be implemented. While this selection procedure may seem fair and that it ensures that those most in need benefit from the programme, there may be other disadvantaged communities with significant HIV incidence and prevalence but who are not serviced by any organisation interested or able to implement such a programme. In such a case a group of adolescents very much in need of such a programme and its intended health benefits may well miss out.

What system of monitoring, evaluation, accountability and redress exists?

Monitoring and evaluation of organisations implementing the GOLD peer education programme is a core component of the programme and an ongoing process throughout. The aim of the monitoring and evaluation process is to monitor organisational progress; track activities conducted; and document information required by the programme's funders (GOLD 2008b). Implementing organisations are required to submit monthly and quarterly progress reports to GOLD's head office. In response, an annual report is prepared by GOLD's head office that provides feedback to all the implementing organisations as to their progress and areas for development or change. Training in monitoring and evaluation is also provided to each implementing organisation as well as templates for all the necessary documentation (GOLD 2008b). The GOLD programme has not been subject to any external evaluation process, nor has it contributed to the published literature regarding the programme and resultant outcomes. Complaints regarding the programme are dealt with at a local level initially but may also be brought to the attention of the organisation's head office (GOLD n.d.).

Conclusion

Neglect of the sexual and reproductive health needs of adolescents in South Africa, and across the globe, has led to poor outcomes for many. Adolescents are shouldering much more than their fair share of ill health in this area. The burden experienced by many adolescents in South Africa today is an example of the vital need for an immediate and appropriate response from health sectors. Campaigns and programmes, such as the GOLD peer education programme, are desperately needed to address the sexual and reproductive health needs of South Africa's adolescent population. Such actions must empower them through knowledge, skills training and community development. Although not explicitly stated in any of the reviewed material, the GOLD programme and curriculum promotes the human rights of young people including their right to enjoy optimal sexual and reproductive health. The programme has yet to be externally evaluated but is extensively evaluated and monitored internally throughout the implementation process. In communities that have services interested and capable of running the GOLD programme a considerable degree of behaviour change amongst those adolescents involved has been shown. Perhaps with the continued and more widely spread implementation of programmes such as GOLD's, the tide may start to turn. The spread of HIV amongst this population group will slow and hopefully reverse. Adolescents in South Africa, and across the globe, may begin to experience a higher level of sexual and reproductive health, both now and into their adulthood.

8 Mid-Day Meal Scheme in Madhya Pradesh

The 'Ruchikar' or Relishing Mid-Day Meal Scheme (RMDMS)

Arjun Singh

Human rights refer to the norms that are internationally recognised and equally applicable to people all over the world. Included in these rights is the right to health, i.e. the right to the highest attainable standard of health (Braveman and Gruskin 2003b). Almost all countries are party to at least one treaty that encompasses rights related to health, and this means that it is the responsibility of the governments of those countries to ensure that their populations are enabled to achieve better health by providing them with conditions that help in realization of the right to health (Braveman and Gruskin 2003a; Gruskin *et al.* 2007). One of the ways through which governments try to fulfil this responsibility is by initiating various policies or programmes. One such programme initiated by the Indian government is the National Programme of Nutritional Support to Primary Education (NP-NSPE) or the Mid-Day Meal Scheme (MDMS) which is intended to give an overall boost to universalisation of primary education (GoI 2005 and Education for All in India 2010) via provision of noon (or mid-day) meals for school-going children in classes 1–5 in all government primary schools. When launched in 1995, some state governments were reluctant to implement it. However, sustained campaigning by the People's Union for Civil Liberties (PUCL) to ensure that the right to food is seen as a corollary of the fundamental right to life as per article 21 of the Indian Constitution (PUCL 2010; Mathiharan 2003), and subsequent Supreme Court orders on the right to food case whereby it has linked the right to food to the right to health as per interpretation of article 47 of the Indian constitution, have effectively put the onus on the central government to ensure that no school-going child remains hungry (Right to Food India 2010).

In this chapter, a human rights analysis of MDMS, implemented in the Indian state of Madhya Pradesh and known as the 'Ruchikar' or Relishing Mid-Day Meal Scheme (RMDMS), is presented using the seven-stage approach to ascertain the extent to which it has been successful, especially with focus on whether it has fostered the realization of human rights of its target population through provision of mid-day meals in schools.

Background

In the world today, the number of chronically hungry children is estimated to be 400 million and out of these one child is dying every six seconds (Chettiparamb 2009).

According to the World Food Programme, the number of underweight children in developing countries is 146 million or 25 per cent of the total children in these countries (Chettiparamb 2009). This is the reason why provision of free-of-cost meals in schools should be given the highest importance for enabling the overall development of their capabilities to fight hunger and to overcome it (Chettiparamb 2009). Along with contributing to the eradication of extreme hunger and poverty, mid-day meals can also help achieve universalisation of primary education and help promote gender equality (Chettiparamb 2009).

The Indian context

In India, the genesis of the Mid-Day Meal Scheme (MDMS) can be traced back to 1925, when the erstwhile municipal corporation of Madras (now Chennai) introduced a Mid-Day Meal programme targeting disadvantaged children (Vencatesan 2008). Later, in the early 1960s, the meals were supplemented with some milk and bread, and the programme was also introduced by other states of Kerala, Pondicherry (now Puducherry) and Gujarat (Vencatesan 2008). In the 1990s, the programme was started by eight more states using their own resources. The success of this initiative led the Indian government to launch it on a nationwide scale in 1995 as the National Programme of Nutritional Support to Primary Education (NP-NSPE) or the Mid-Day Meal Scheme (MDMS) (Vencatesan 2008; GoI 2005). The programme has been revised twice since then. In the 2004 revision, 300 calories and 8–12g of protein were mandated to be provided to each child and consideration was made for providing food to drought-prone areas even during the vacations (Vencatesan 2008; GoI 2005; Education for All in India 2010). The 2006 revision mandated an increase in the amounts of calories and proteins in cooked meals and that the cooked meal had to have a recommended dosage of micronutrients (Vencatesan 2008). This was an important step as micronutrient-fortified food can reverse the effect of most micronutrient deficiencies and prevent the occurrence of health problems that can affect the growth and development of children (Osei et al. 2008, 2010). Other changes included making the Food Corporation of India (FCI) responsible for supplying food-grains to support this increase (Vencatesan 2008), and linking the programme to other programmes that were going on at the time like the 'Sarva Shiksha Abhiyan' (the Universal Literacy Programme), 'Swajaldhara' (the accelerated rural water supply programme) and the National Rural Health Mission (Vencatesan 2008). Chettiparamb (2009) contends that direct provisioning, geographical stability in price and heightened access are ensured using such an approach.

Madhya Pradesh was one of the first states to implement the MDMS in 1995 (Jain and Shah 2005). By 2003, it had been implemented throughout the state. Other states that had fully implemented this programme by 2003 included Rajasthan, Gujarat, Chhattisgarh, Andhra Pradesh, Karnataka, Kerala, Tamil Nadu, Tripura and Sikkim (NFI 2009). However, malnutrition is still responsible for one out of every two child deaths in Madhya Pradesh. The state has the highest rate of infant mortality and the lowest life expectancy in India, and amongst children less than 5 years old more than 60 per cent are malnourished, with the situation being worse in the tribal areas (Samvad et al. 2009). Inadequate budgetary allocation and shortcomings in coordination and convergence among departments involved in implementing the MDMS and little or no participation from the community have made tackling malnutrition the biggest challenge before the state government (Samvad et al. 2009).

Stage 1: the specific intended purpose of MDMS

Purpose and target population

According to Gostin and Mann (1994), it is essential to have a clear understanding of the purpose of the public health policy or programme. MDMS was introduced on a nationwide basis in all government primary schools for children in classes 1–5 with two major purposes. The first was to boost universalisation of primary education by directing efforts to enhance enrolment, retention and class attendance (GoI 2005; Education for All in India 2010) and to increase access to education so that these children are not pushed or forced to work at an early age (Saxena 2002). The second purpose was to improve the nutritional levels among these children by introducing cooked mid-day meals within two years of the launch (GoI 2005; Education for All in India 2010) and thereby bring down the incidence of malnutrition (Saxena 2002).

Since these two major purposes were uniform for all states where MDMS was implemented, Madhya Pradesh and RMDMS were no exception. Moreover, MDMS also made a provision for appointing cooks from scheduled castes and scheduled tribes (Jain and Shah 2005). Thus, it also provided for employment of people from the disadvantaged classes. As noted earlier, MDMS was first revised in 2004 and under this revision it came to be known as RMDMS in Madhya Pradesh. However, the two major purposes remained unchanged. All further analysis will be provided against the backdrop of this first revision.

Mechanisms and interventions

In addition to getting central assistance, Madhya Pradesh also set up the appropriate infrastructure for implementing the scheme. Central assistance included free supply of food-grains from the nearest FCI warehouse, subsidies for transport of food-grains to schools and increased assistance for cooking which included bearing the cost of ingredients, fuel and wages for the agency responsible for cooking (GoI 2005). Monetary assistance included provision for construction of a kitchen-cum-store and for replacement of kitchen devices (GoI 2005).

The role of state and local bodies is also important. In Madhya Pradesh, the MDMS is devolved to village councils (Gram Panchayats) (Chettiparambil-Rajan 2007). Thus in villages of Madhya Pradesh, the financial and administrative responsibility for implementing the MDMS is primarily with the village councils. Grants linked to central government schemes such as the Sampoorna Gramin Rozgar Yojana (SGRY), which aims to provide food security and improve nutritional levels in rural areas (DRDA 2010), and moolbhoot rashi (or untied grants) devolved by the State

Finance Commission are the two main sources of funds for the village councils. However, through local tax revenue, the councils can also raise their own resources (Afridi 2005). Supervision and implementation of RMDMS are expected to be carried out by the Village Education Committee and the Parent Teacher Association (PTA) of the schools (Afridi 2005).

Stage 2

An impartial and careful examination of various facts, expert opinion and consultation with affected groups is the way to ascertain effectiveness (Gostin and Mann 1994). An evaluation of RMDMS was done in seventy government primary schools in six districts of Anuppur, Khandwa, Mandla, Shivpuri, Sidhi and Tikamgarh in Madhya Pradesh by Jain and Shah (2005). The findings of this evaluation revealed a number of shortcomings, as well as positive features.

The first of the shortcomings was meal quality. Food quality is an important predictor of children's participation in school meals (Lülfs-Baden and Spiller 2009; Lülfs-Baden *et al.* 2008). According to Jain and Shah (2005), there were variations in meal quality due to factors like the price of the ingredients used in making the meals. In some districts, with the scarce availability of vegetables other than onions, potatoes and pumpkins, meals were sometimes watery.

A second area of shortcoming was in infrastructure and systems. A proper kitchen was found in only 7 per cent of the schools surveyed, and there was also no permanent space for cooking, with most of it being done in either a temporary shed or in an open space in the school premises or even in the cook's home. This meant a compromise on cleanliness and accountability and a clear violation of the Supreme Court's order pertaining to the right to food case (Jain and Shah 2005).

Thirdly, the evaluation identified some caste discrimination. Not only are dalits, i.e. the very poor and disadvantaged people of the state, not appointed as cooks in most schools, but the food cooked by them is not eaten by many, especially by upper caste children (Jain and Shah 2005).

A final shortcoming was the burden on teachers. There being no separate arrangement for meal management, teachers had to spend extra time on work related to preparing the meal, which resulted in their being unable to give adequate time for teaching (Jain and Shah 2005).

There were also a number of positive findings. First, in relation to meal regularity, when asked whether cooked meals were provided daily, almost 90 per cent of the teachers and cooks answered that they were, with this percentage being slightly lower for parents (Jain and Shah 2005). For meal quality, although a tenth of parents found the meal below acceptable standards, there were no serious complaints from any of the parents, teachers and cooks about any child suffering from a serious illness after consuming a mid-day meal (Jain and Shah 2005). O'Brien (2008) contends that, although meal standards may be challenging to implement locally, meals cooked according to such standards help reduce both inequalities in health and the burden of chronic diseases like cancer, diabetes, coronary heart disease and osteoporosis.

PTAs were entrusted with the responsibility of implementing RMDMS rather than village councils. The non-official head of the PTA and the teacher in-charge jointly administered funds for it and developed elaborate inspection and monitoring protocols. Active participation of both parents and teachers has been critical to this empowerment of PTAs and the overall effectiveness of RMDMS (Jain and Shah 2005). Drèze and Kingdon (2001) are of the opinion that cooperation between parents and teachers has a positive influence on school participation and/or academic achievement. For example, in New Delhi, parents are invited to schools to be an integral part of tasting and approving the cooked food. Indeed, Gostin and Mann (1994) contend that health programmes should incorporate the principle of informed consent as suggested by legal and ethical standards. According to Rosoff (1981), every person has, in relation to her health and wellbeing, the right to make appropriate decisions. Thus this step ensured that the scheme had endorsement and informed consent from the parents (Diwan 2009).

Overall the evaluation identified tremendous approval for the scheme. Despite the drawbacks mentioned, the scheme got overwhelming approval from almost 96 per cent of parents, with only 4 per cent of parents in Anuppur and Tikamgarh disapproving on grounds of very poor meal quality and quantity. Overall, most parents felt that it had become easier for them to send their children to school and children became more interested in their studies and took them more seriously (Jain and Shah 2005). Most teachers also voiced the same opinion and indicated that the scheme should be continued due to its positive effects on student enrolment, attendance and retention (Jain and Shah 2005). Children too liked the 'ruchikar' meal and stopped going home to have their meal. Thus the meal improved their retention. On the whole, a 15 per cent increase in enrolment was registered, whereas the increase for girls was even higher at 19 per cent and 21 per cent for girls from scheduled castes/tribes. These increases were seen despite significant inter-district and inter-community variations (Jain and Shah 2005). The most dramatic rise in enrolment was for children from scheduled castes/tribes (41 per cent) suggesting that, for people who suffer relatively greater deprivation, it is the meal that matters the most (Jain and Shah 2005).

Finally, in terms of cost effectiveness, according to Afridi (2005), protein and calorie deficiency of participants was reduced by 100 per cent and almost 30 per cent respectively for as little as 3 cents. Moreover, with a very low per pupil per day cost (which varies between 0.50 and 5 rupees depending on the quality of the cooked meal), the scheme had the potential to alter trade-offs in parents' decisions regarding the schooling of their children. As it promised improved nutritional status for the participating child, it increased the benefits of schooling and this lowered the opportunity cost of attending school (Afridi 2005).

The RMDMS positively impacted student enrolment, attendance and retention. It also had a socialization and egalitarian value as children learnt to sit together and share the meal (Drèze and Goyal 2003; PIB 2010). According to Singh (2008), the effects of MDMS on learning are encouraging and mid-day meals form a valuable safety net against nutritional deprivation. By boosting female school attendance more than male school attendance (Drèze and Goyal 2003) and employing more female cooks, RMDMS helped enhance gender equity (PIB 2010) and also freed the girl child from her traditional caretaker role in the family (Vencatesan 2008). So it can be said that, as RMDMS produced the outcomes it intended via provision of RMDMS, it was appropriate, accurate and effective.

Stage 3: impacts on rights

Gostin and Mann (1994) contend that policies which are well conceived are those that target the people in need, and awareness of whether they are over- or under-inclusive sensitises the public health community to concerns regarding human rights. Thus in this stage, a more specific analysis of RMDMS is carried out.

Is RMDMS discriminatory in any way?

It was noted earlier that there was a reluctance to appoint dalits as cooks, and refusal by upper caste children to consume food cooked by them. Moreover, some upper caste children even refused to sit next to lower caste children while having their meals (Jain and Shah 2005). This does not reflect any inherent or intended design flaw or discrimination in the programme but only indicates the prevalence of the caste system in certain parts of Madhya Pradesh.

Over- and under-inclusion

Since MDMS is conducted in all government primary schools throughout the country, children belonging to less privileged families who study in private schools are inevitably excluded from it, irrespective of the state MDMS is implemented in, including Madhya Pradesh. However, about 4 per cent of private schools which are central government-aided are covered by it (Singh 2008). This may represent under-inclusion, but according to Gostin and Mann (1994), such under-inclusiveness may only indicate the public health problem and priorities of a country rather than any discrimination. On the other hand, by 2003, MDMS had been implemented throughout Madhya Pradesh (NFI 2009). This indicates that all districts, irrespective of whether children were malnourished or illiterate or not, were covered by the scheme. In the opinion of Swaminathan (2008), inclusion of beneficiaries who are not eligible for programmes that target the hungry may result in higher financial or fiscal programme costs. This, however, is in accordance with the goal of the National Programme of Nutritional Support to Primary Education of giving an overall boost to universalisation of primary education (GoI 2005; Education for All in India 2010) in all government primary schools.

Rights impacted positively

The success of RMDMS indicated that through provision of mid-day meals in schools, the problem of malnutrition and low class attendance had been addressed to a large extent and this has ensured the realization of the right to food of children in these areas. Here, it is noteworthy that the Supreme Court has held that, since India is party to the International Covenant on Civil and Political Rights (ICCPR) and the International Covenant on Economic, Social and Cultural Rights (ICESCR), the interpretation of article 21 of the Indian constitution, which gives protection to life and liberty of all citizens, has to be made in accordance with international law (Mathiharan 2003). Moreover, the Supreme Court put the onus on the state to create means and conditions for improving the health of its population by referring to article 47 of the constitution, according to which raising the level of nutrition and standard of living, and improving public health, are duties of the state (GoI 2008). Thus, it linked the right to food to the right to health. With this backdrop, it is clear that RMDMS positively impacted not only the right to health and thus right to life as per interpretation of articles 47 and 21 of the constitution, but also the right to education under article 26 of the Universal Declaration of Human Rights (UDHR) and article 13 of ICESCR. By gainfully employing many people as cooks, it also positively impacted article 23 of UDHR, articles 6 and 7 of ICESCR, and article 41 of the constitution which guarantees the right to work and education (GoI 2008). RMDMS also positively impacted article 39(f) of the constitution which grants protection of children against exploitation. As there are links between right to food and right to health, a positive impact on the former can be said to also impact the latter positively. Thus in essence, the right to health under article 12 of ICESCR has been positively impacted.

Research opinion about alternatives

There is no evidence of RMDMS being coercive, punitive, restrictive or not being humane according to its review done by Jain and Shah (2005) and Afridi (2005). Although discrimination may be carried out by some people using unfair means, which may include coercion or enforcing some restrictions, etc., this is not a feature of RMDMS as a means of realising its objectives.

Stage 4: restrictions of rights?

Gostin and Mann (1994) are of the view that the best health strategies are those which respect a person's inherent dignity. The reviews of RMDMS by Jain and Shah (2005) and Afridi (2005) make no mention of whether it was compulsory to participate in the scheme or that its implementation necessitated compulsion. Thus, it is not possible to ascertain whether RMDMS was restrictive, coercive and punitive. No further analysis in this stage is therefore possible.

This also means that stage 5, which involves ascertaining whether any restriction on human rights by a policy or programme is justified according to the Siracusa principles, is not applicable.

Stage 6: implementation

In this section, some factors that have hindered the implementation of RMDMS are examined. In Tikamgarh, the PTA was non-functional. Due to this, there was no monitoring of RMDMS by teachers and parents (Jain and Shah 2005). Where a PTA existed, the extent of parental participation determined both the effectiveness of the PTA and proper monitoring and implementation of RMDMS. In Khandwa, Mandla and Sidhi, and in Dewas, only 35 per cent and 15 per cent of parents surveyed were active participants in monitoring and implementation respectively, and consequently, RMDMS suffered (Jain and Shah 2005).

Another problem in implementation was delay in delivery of food-grains. In more than 50 per cent of schools, food-grain delivery was delayed (Jain and Shah 2005). This was due to problems with the targeted public distribution system that had been put in place (Saxena 2002). Meals could not be prepared in sufficient quantity as a result. There were also problems with poorly developed supporting infrastructure: improper kitchens, lack of facilities for drinking water, inadequate number of utensils for cooking, eating, storage and serving were major infrastructural shortcomings (Jain and Shah 2005).

Finally, the absence of separate meal management meant that teachers were unduly burdened as they had to teach and look after monitoring and implementation of RMDMS simultaneously (Jain and Shah 2005). It is clear that there were a few infrastructural problems that hindered the implementation of RMDMS. It is also evident, however, that these did not apply equally in all districts or schools surveyed. For example, a non-functional PTA was seen only in Tikamgarh, and food-grain delivery was on time in nearly 50 per cent of schools.

Stage 7: monitoring, evaluation, accountability

In the last stage in the analysis of RMDMS, the mechanisms set up for monitoring, evaluation, provision of information and grievance redress are discussed. These are laid down in instructions given by the central government. The Department of School Education and Literacy, Ministry of Human Resource Development, has set up a comprehensive and elaborate mechanism according to which representatives of village councils/village meetings and members of various local committees will monitor the scheme on a daily basis and will also look at whether there is social and gender equity (GoI 2005). According to Chettiparambil-Rajan (2007), the MDMS is devolved to village councils which also have the financial and administrative responsibility of implementing the MDMS. Accordingly, the village councils have the primary authority to administer RMDMS, and PTAs ensure proper monitoring and implementation (Jain and Shah 2005).

It has also been made mandatory to provide, as per the Right to Information Act, information about quality of food-grains received, their utilization, daily menu, rosters of members of the community who are involved in the scheme, etc., to ensure that there is accountability and transparency in the running of the scheme in all schools and centres where it is being implemented (GoI 2005). According to the central government, states and Union Territories (UTs) are required to develop a dedicated mechanism for public grievance redress, which should be widely publicised and made easily accessible (GoI 2005). However, there is no mention of such a mechanism in reviews done by Jain and Shah (2005) and Afridi (2005).

Conclusion

It is clear that by providing mid-day meals, RMDMS gave an opportunity to children of poor and marginalised families to be healthy and created a valuable safety net against nutritional deprivation. It also provided them with facilities to develop in a healthy manner and in conditions of freedom and dignity. According to Bambas (2005), the fact that everyone deserves to be treated with dignity is one of the most fundamental human rights. In this light, RMDMS proved to be very successful. Moreover, by employing dalits as cooks, it tried to ensure that people belonging to the disadvantaged classes were provided with equal opportunities in employment. Thus RMDMS also provided for a fair and equitable deployment of resources and tried to create equal opportunities for health by bringing down, to the lowest level possible, health differentials. Moreover, the Supreme Court's orders in the right to food case strongly impress that it is the state's responsibility to ensure that the means to improve health of the population, especially of the vulnerable, are put in place for the promotion of health and health opportunities, and that a proactive approach taken by the judiciary can go a long way in addressing issues or problems that impact health equity and human rights.

9 Tobacco Prevention Strategy in Styria, Austria

A human rights analysis

Michaela Adamowitsch

The purpose of this chapter is to present a human rights analysis of the Tobacco Prevention Strategy (TPS) Styria. Styria is one of nine Austrian federal states and has currently approximately 1.2 million inhabitants (Statistics Austria 2010a). Human rights can be used as a framework for the interrogation of the civil, political, economic, social and cultural environments people live in and how these environments have a direct effect on people's health status (Gruskin and Tarantola 2001). Consequently, the consideration of human rights can also be used as an approach for designing, implementing and evaluating health policies and programmes (Gruskin and Tarantola 2001). In this chapter a seven-stage approach to human rights analysis will be used.

Stage 1: what is the specific intended purpose of the strategy?

The development of the Tobacco Prevention Strategy (TPS) Styria started in 2005 with an implementation period of five years, 2005–10. In the meantime two reports were published in 2007 and 2008 and are publicly available on the internet (Koller 2007; Fernandez and Koller 2008). Up to early 2011 no annual reports for 2009 and 2010 could be retrieved online. Selected and more recent information on TPS activities and news was also sourced on the TPS homepage (www.rauchfrei-dabei. at; only in German language). The specific intended purpose of the strategy is to prevent and reduce tobacco consumption in Styria and to thereby reduce associated adverse health effects (Fernandez and Koller 2008). Four general aims have been designed for the TPS Styria (Koller 2007):

- Aim 1: Fewer people start smoking;
- Aim 2: More people quit smoking;
- Aim 3: Protection of people from the consequences of passive smoking;
- Aim 4: Improvement of the level of information regarding the consequences of smoking and passive smoking and modification of mindsets and attitudes in the population (towards tobacco consumption and passive smoking).

To evaluate these aims, principles for health promotion planning can be applied, as the overall purpose of the Styrian strategy, generally speaking, is to promote health. Aims 1 and 2 focus on health-related behaviour; while aim 3 focuses on the environment, and aim 4 focuses on individuals/groups (according to the examples given in Tones and Green 2004; Koller 2007). The aims are formulated broadly as they do not mention specific target groups; instead they address the entire population of Styria. Although being not population-specific, they seem to meet the general purpose of aims (Tones and Green 2004): they are useful to lead actions and to build a shared understanding among stakeholders of what they want to attain. This chapter focuses on the analysis of only two of the aims in detail, aims 2 and 4. Table 9.1 shows the objectives corresponding to each of the four aims.

The suitability of objectives can be appraised by applying the SMART-criteria: objectives should be: specific, measurable, achievable, realistic and time limited (Tones and Green 2004). The objectives of the selected aims fulfil the requirement to describe them more specifically. They mention specific target groups within the Styrian population, and the objectives of aim 2 are time limited, as opposed to the objectives for aim 4. Only a few of them are highly specific (such as 2.1 and 2.2). Objective 2.8 and those for aim 4 are formulated rather vaguely and may thereby be difficult to measure. The objectives seem to be theoretically achievable, but the remaining question is whether they are all achievable in the chosen time period (if determined). The fact that the list of the objectives ends with 'etcetera' creates the impression that the objectives are not complete or not completely settled, which is not in accordance with the recommendations for health promotion objectives.

A strength of the strategy is that the aims and objectives are based on an extensive baseline evaluation ('Smoking in Styria'), conducted in 2006, and commissioned by the two major stakeholders, the Styrian Landtag (parliament) and the main Styrian health insurance company (STGKK). The relevant results of the evaluation are published in the annual reports, where they are discussed separately for every aim (Koller 2007; Fernandez and Koller 2008). Areas for intervention have also been based on the findings of this evaluation (see Table 9.2). According to Tones and Green (2004), this sort of in-depth analysis of underlying determinants of an issue helps to define the aims of a strategy, as it allows the identification of relevant influences on health status, important target groups and their characteristics, stakeholders, as well as possible approaches for interventions.

The strategy as a whole sets out to cover children in childcare centres and schools, adolescents (out-of-school), people in municipalities all over Styria, people working in the health sector and people in the workplace. All services are free of cost except 'Smoke-free seminars' (one-off payment of €30) and access is not limited to any population group (except the age limitation for the adolescents' seminar). Evaluation showed that the age of participants in the 'Smoke-free' programmes ranged between 25 and 70 years.

Stage 2: what are the ways and the extent to which the strategy may impact positively and negatively on health?

The form of the intervention areas and activities can be regarded as appropriate and accurate as they have been established not only on the basis of a baseline evaluation

Table 9.1 Aims and objectives of TPS Styria

	Aim	Timeframe	Objectives
1	Fewer people start smoking	10 years	1. Smoking initiation age is raised to age 15 2. Smoking rate amongst adolescents is reduced by 1% per year
2	More people quit smoking	10 years (objectives 1 to 3) 3 years (objectives 4 to 9)	1. Reduction of smoking prevalence of men by 2% per year 2. Reduction of smoking prevalence of women by 1% per year 3. Reduced number of heavy smokers 4. Existence of age specific and gender specific services/activities 5. Availability of sufficient financial and personal resources to existing institutions offering new services 6. Increased number of people who quit smoking successfully 7. Increased number of smokers who want to quit smoking 8. Smokers who wish to quit receive adequate support for it 9. Reduced number of years people smoke before quitting
3	Protection of people from the consequences of passive smoking	3 years	1. Insurance of particular protection for children, adolescents and pregnant women 2. Change of people's consciousness; existence of mutual understanding 3. The population is informed about adverse health effects of passive smoking 4. People who are exposed to passive smoking in their workplace perceive this as pestering and demand smoke-free workplaces
3	Improvement of the level of information regarding the consequences of smoking and passive smoking and modification of mindsets and attitudes in the population (towards tobacco consumption and passive smoking)	–	1. Parents are able to impart skills to their children that reduce tobacco consumption 2. Educators and people working with children and adolescents are able to impart skills that reduce tobacco consumption 3. Changes in knowledge, mindsets and attitudes 4. Adolescents and children grow up in a surrounding that can prevent the consumption of tobacco 5. Pregnant women and young parents are informed about harmful consequences of tobacco consumption 6. Medical practitioners, other healthcare professionals and people working in advisory centres are able to pass on information correctly 7. Medical practitioners, other healthcare professionals and people working in advisory centres are aware of the importance of handing on information 8. Policy makers, politicians and media are aware of the importance of the issue and provide information in an effective way

Source: adapted from Bachinger 2005, as cited in Fernandez & Koller (2008: 9)

Table 9.2 Selected aims and associated interventions and actions of TPS Styria

Aim	Areas for intervention and single actions

2. More people quit smoking	• *Education and training*
	  • Education of 'dehabituation experts' for the 'Smoke-free in 6 weeks program'; some of them receive further education to become multipliers on the health care sector
	  • Advanced training of lecturers from Styrian health and nursing schools, as well as for school physicians and Styrian pharmacists.
	• *Promotion for quitting smoking targeting adolescents*
	  • 'Take control' – free seminars for 16 to 25 year-olds
	• *Counselling and dehabituation*
	  • 'Smoke-free in 6 weeks' – free group sessions; also offered at workplaces
	  • Web-based program for quitting smoking
	  • Individual free counselling of smokers offered by STGKK
	• *Providing information and raising public awareness*
	  • Free telephone helpline (in addition to the 'Austrian smoke-hotline')
	  • Brochure 'Smoke-free during pregnancy'
	  • STGKK promotes intensification of patient motivation to quit through physicians
	  • Special promotion month in pharmacies

4. Improvement of the level of information regarding the consequences of smoking and passive smoking	• *Providing information and raising public awareness*
	  • Homepage launched in 2007
	  • Campaign 'Vitamin instead of nicotine' on World-non-smoker-day
	  • Public relation (marketing for offered programs, e.g. in newspapers, at events, in medical clinics; press relations; development of a PR concept 2009/2010)
	  • Networking (organisation of expert conference; symposium for out-of-school work with youth; sending quarterly newsletters)

Source: Fernandez and Koller 2008

but also on a review in the area of tobacco prevention that has been compiled in a strategy document prior to the development of the TPS Styria ('Recommendations for a Tobacco Prevention Strategy for Styria', unpublished; Bachinger 2005, as cited in Fernandez and Koller 2008: 9). The recommendations in this document are based on the World Health Organization's publication for the Framework Convention on Tobacco Control (WHO 2003b), on the European Strategy for Tobacco Control (EURO 2002), on strategies of countries that have successfully implemented and evaluated tobacco strategies and on an analysis of potential stakeholders and interested parties in Styria (Koller 2007). TPS Styria is based on findings from studies that showed that drug-preventive strategies are effective in significantly improving quality of life in populations (Brühler and Kröger 2006; Canning *et al.* 2004; Jones *et al.* 2006; Shin 2001, as cited in Fernandez and Koller 2008: 9; Hawks *et al.* 2002).

Obtaining informed consent from participants in strategy activities is not an issue in regard to the TPS Styria as the participation in any intervention action is fully voluntary. The use of voluntary non-smoking strategies is supported in an article on new directions for tobacco control by Jacobson and Banerjee (2005). However, Fernandez and Koller (2008) stress in their report that a sustainable reduction of tobacco consumption in the population would demand an additional strategy on the national level, which would imply the enactment of more extensive tobacco laws, raising of the tobacco tax and the reinforcement of actions against cigarette smuggling.

The evaluation of health impacts of the TPS Styria is difficult. The report from 2008 says that a time period of at least ten years will be required to reach the health-promoting strategy aims, as results of health-promoting programmes are usually only achievable in the long term (Fernandez and Koller 2008). This is inconsistent with the timeframe for action that is stated later in the 2008 report; see Table 9.1. Evaluation of TPS activities and programmes and their results is also difficult because they are influenced by numerous unpredictable external factors at both the individual and social level (Fernandez and Koller 2008). Furthermore, measuring the prevalence rate of tobacco consumption in the adult population to determine the effectiveness of tobacco preventive interventions is not practicable as there are currently no survey tools that can deliver reliable prevalence rates (Uhl et al. 2009).

Consequently, only results of short-term outcomes of some TPS activities are available so far; evaluation of those will form the basis for the final evaluation after the initiative finishes in 2010: the report from 2008 includes details of the 'Take control' and 'Smoke-free in 6 weeks' programme evaluation. Results show that more girls than boys completed the four-week 'Take control' seminar, and that smoking behaviour could be reduced: more than half of the participants reduced their cigarette consumption by at least 50 per cent, from data collected at the end of the seminar (Fernandez and Koller 2008). Cigarette consumption increased in ten adolescents (out of a total of 115): four of those said that the seminar did not work for them while the other six adolescents had already very low smoking rates prior to the seminar and intended to quit in the near future (Fernandez and Koller 2008). Only forty-four adolescents could be interviewed in the six-month follow-up survey; smoking rates were above those measured after the seminar but not as high as initial rates (Fernandez and Koller 2008). Altogether 979 people participated in the 105 'Smoke-free in 6 weeks' groups (thirty-two in workplaces); this programme is based on the manual by Batra and Buchkremer (2004, as cited in Koller 2007: 30), which conforms with guidelines for tobacco dehabituation. Since 2008, three-month follow-up care via telephone is also available. Repeated evaluation showed abstinence rates from smoking of 25–35 per cent at twelve-month follow-up and found participants to be highly satisfied with the programme (Fernandez and Koller 2008).

No other evaluations of TPS activities are available from annual reports. More recent information on evaluation results, although only in a highly condensed form, is available from the TPS newsletter for September 2010. According to the findings of public opinion polls, conducted in 2006 and 2009, the proportion of people who are informed about adverse health effects of passive smoking increased by 2.5 per cent; more than half of Styrian non-smokers who know about TPS services say that they now tell smokers not to smoke in the presence of children; also, more smokers say that they try to avoid smoking when children are nearby; Styrians also remembered awareness-raising campaigns, for example, eight out of ten people recalled a poster showing a 4-month-old boy asking 'Am I already allowed to smoke?' (VIVID 2010). Furthermore, 90 per cent of the population wanted TPS strategies to be continued; 'Smoke-free in 6 weeks' group sessions increased from twenty-five sessions in 2007 to 101 sessions (815 participants) in 2009, now being offered almost all over Styria, and eighty-six people were trained to become 'dehabituation-experts'. Between February 2007 and May 2010 300 people working in the health sector were trained on tobacco issues to become disseminators; guidelines for tobacco prevention in schools as well as for out-of-school have been developed and are currently being tested; topics around tobacco were integrated into further education of kindergarten workers and teachers, as well as into parents' evenings; a children's book was developed and sent to all kindergartens, health practitioners, paediatricians and gynaecologists in Styria (VIVID 2010).

Evidence for other intervention activities is also available from Hopkins *et al.* (2001), who conducted an extensive review of interventions for the reduction of tobacco consumption. These authors found, inter alia, strong evidence for the effectiveness of telephone cessation support that is implemented together with other interventions (e.g. educational strategies) in the clinical or community setting; 796 Styrians used the helpline of the TPS in 2008 (Fernandez and Koller 2008). Sufficient evidence also exists for health care provider reminder systems and their effectiveness in enhancing the provision of advice for quitting to smokers (Hopkins *et al.* 2001); this justifies the STGKK's promotion of patient-motivation intensification to quit through physicians. Strong evidence also exists that multi-component health care system interventions, including a provider reminder system and provider education programme, successfully enhance providers' provision of advice for quitting and smoking cessation; education of smokers at the same time showed additional effectiveness (Hopkins *et al.* 2001). No research evidence could be found for the existence of any potential negative health effects of a tobacco prevention strategy.

Out of the range of recommendations given in the strategy document created in 2006, only those initiatives have been chosen for implementation that were suitable in regard to financial, personal and structural resources of the TPS strategy at federal state level (Fernandez and Koller 2008).

Stage 3: what and whose rights are impacted positively and negatively by the strategy?

The purpose of the Tobacco Prevention Strategy in Styria has several human rights implications, especially in regard to the right to health, the rights of children and women's rights. These three areas have been identified by Dresler and Marks (2006) in their article on the formation of a human right to tobacco control.

The right to health

Research evidence shows that numerous diseases are caused by smoking: coronary heart disease, peripheral vascular disease, stroke, multiple forms of cancer, chronic obstructive pulmonary disease, and peptic ulcer disease; smoking during pregnancy has also negative impacts on foetal and neonatal development (Fagerström 2002). Consequently, the TPS Styria impacts positively on the right to health, which is implied in article 25 of the Universal Declaration of Human Rights (UN General Assembly 1948), in article 12 of the International Covenant on Economic, Social and Cultural Rights (ICESCR) (UN General Assembly 1966a), and in the General Comment 14 (GC 14) (CESCR 2000). GC 14 comments on article 12.2(b) of the ICESCR (the right to healthy natural and workplace environments) that the article comprises the 'prevention and reduction of the population's exposure to harmful substances such as ... harmful chemicals or other detrimental environmental conditions that directly or indirectly impact upon human health' and that it 'discourages ... the use of tobacco' (CESCR 2000: para 15). Furthermore, General Comment 14 (CESCR 2000) elaborates on article 12.2(c) of the ICESCR (the right to prevention, treatment and control of diseases) that it 'requires the establishment of prevention and education programmes for behaviour-related health concerns' (CESCR 2000: para 16). Intervention areas of TPS Styria promote the right to a healthy environment, healthy and safe work conditions, and accessible health education and information as outlined in General Comment 14: almost all objectives for aims 2 and 4 promote, directly or indirectly, healthy environments, including the work environment (in respect to active and passive smoking); and objective 2.8 and all objectives of aim 4 (increase of knowledge) address access to health education and information. Objectives 2.4, 2.5 and 2.8 fulfil the requirements of paragraph 16 of GC 14.

TPS intervention activities are also in accordance with paragraph 18 of GC 14 (CESCR 2000), regarding non-discrimination and equal treatment: 'the vulnerable members of society must be protected by the adoption of relatively low-cost targeted programmes'. The report of 2008 explains that it is important for TPS-initiators that the activities are low-threshold services to allow a broad population reach: activities are free of cost (except for the small one-off payment for adult group sessions) and thereby accessible to population groups of low socio-economic background (Fernandez and Koller 2008). This is especially important as population groups of lower educational or occupational levels in Styria have a higher share of smokers (Bachinger 2005, as cited in Fernandez and Koller 2008: 9).

However, Backman et al. (2008) identified ten more grounds of discrimination in UN treaties in addition to socio-economic status: age, sex, ethnic origin, age, disability, language, religion, national origin, political or other opinion and property. Out of these, TPS Styria could be discriminatory towards population groups that live in Austria but do not speak German fluently. Nine per cent of the Styrian population are migrants (90 of 1,000 inhabitants are first-generation immigrants); 24,400 persons with a citizenship from former Yugoslavia and 5,500 persons with Turkish citizenship lived in Styria in 2009 (Statistics Austria 2010b). While the brochure for parents is available online in Turkish, English and in Serbo-Croatian languages on the homepage, no hints could be found for the existence of any other material in other languages. The only non-German service that could be located was a group session offered in English which was announced to begin in October

2010 (VIVID 2010). If this is the case, this could be regarded as a violation of the International Convention on the Elimination of All Forms of Racial Discrimination (UN General Assembly 1965). Consequently, TPS Styria may bear some risk of under-inclusion of these population groups. Over-inclusion of people is not an issue in regard to TPS Styria as the intent is to address the entire population, which may lead to a change in social norms regarding the use of tobacco.

Rights of children

TPS Styria is also supportive in regard to the right to health, the rights to information and education for children and 'the right of every child to a standard of living adequate for the child's physical, mental, spiritual, moral and social development' (article 27) that is covered in the Convention on the Rights of the Child (CRC) (UN General Assembly 1989). TPS also meets what is demanded in paragraph 23 of GC 14 (CESCR 2000), which urges states to 'provide a safe and supportive environment for adolescents, that ensures the opportunity to participate in decisions affecting their health, to build life-skills, to acquire appropriate information, to receive counselling and to negotiate the health-behaviour choices they make'.

Women's rights

TPS Styria is furthermore supportive for women's right to healthy and safe work conditions and access to health care, including information and counselling, as covered in the Convention on the Elimination of All Forms of Discrimination Against Women (CEDAW) (UN General Assembly 1979).

Stage 4: does the strategy necessitate the restriction of human rights?

TPS Styria does not necessitate the restriction of human rights in respect of aims 2 and 4.

Stage 5: if so, have the criteria/preconditions to restrict rights been met?

Not applicable, see stage 4 above.

Stage 6: are health and other relevant structures and services capable of effectively implementing the strategy?

According to the annual reports (Koller 2007; Fernandez and Koller 2008), TPS seems to be well-thought-out and the implementation seems to be professionally organised. Major Styrian institutions (the Landtag Styria and the main health insurance company, STGKK), who are the main initiators of TPS, ensure that the resources (personnel, financial) for the implementation are available: in 2008,

€661,497 were available as subsidies for the implementation of intervention activities (Fernandez and Koller 2008). The organisational structure of TPS is also clearly set out in the reports: by order of the Landtag Styria, VIVID (Styrian department for the prevention of addiction) is responsible for the implementation of the strategy in the form of yearly projects, and therefore VIVID cooperates with STGKK (Fernandez and Koller 2008). No factors could be identified that might interfere with the strategy implementation.

Stage 7: what system of monitoring, evaluation, accountability and redress exists?

Since 2008, a steering committee has been responsible for decision-making and consequently for monitoring the strategy implementation (Fernandez and Koller 2008). The Swiss Impact Model for Health Promotion is going to be used for the evaluation of TPS after finishing the project in 2010 (Gesundheisförderung Schweiz 2009); the annual reports do not set out who will do the evaluation. The annual reports that have been published so far, as well as other TPS material, are freely available on the internet. All the information used in this chapter in regard to TPS is accessible to every German-speaking person who has access to the internet. None of the TPS information reviewed clearly set out who is accountable in regard to TPS. Contact details that are given in the reports and on the internet are those of VIVID. Project partners such as the STGKK and Landtag Styria are named, although no contact details are provided. It is assumed that any person of those institutions would be available for complaints or feedback from individuals, but as there seems to be no clear system for complaints or feedback it is questionable if complaints/feedback would be effective. No hints could be found for the existence of assistance to different groups who might have difficulty raising any complaints/feedback.

Conclusion

The core elements of TPS Styria comprise awareness-raising amongst all population groups regarding adverse health effects of smoking and passive smoking, the establishment of services for dehabituation all over Styria, and education and training of professionals working in the health and social sectors. From the present human rights analysis, which has been based on current TPS online data and documents, it can be concluded that the Styrian strategy also supports several human rights: the right to health, the rights of children, as well as women's rights. Recommendations that can be drawn from the analysis are that more services and materials could be provided for non-German-speaking inhabitants of Styria; and contact persons, opportunities for feedback and according assistance could be clearly indicated on the homepage and in reports. Altogether, the evidence-based, long-term, multi-method and multi-level approach TPS Styria is based on makes it a good model for tobacco prevention practice and it appears worthwhile to transfer this model to other Austrian federal states.

10 National MindMatters Project

A retrospective human rights analysis

Carmel Treacy

This chapter examines the Australian MindMatters Project from a human rights perspective. It does this, first, by briefly outlining the MindMatters Project, then, using the 'seven-stage' approach to human rights analysis as outlined by Gruskin and Tarantola (2001), the student outcomes of the professional development method will be discussed. This method of examining the project considers how human rights are both supported and weakened through its implementation, drawing on evidence from relevant literature.

Synopsis of MindMatters project

MindMatters is a nationally implemented project in secondary schools in Australia, which aims to promote mental health and wellbeing in students. It was established as a 'whole of school' approach, which is a term implying 'changes in curriculum, policies, structures and partnerships' (Hazell 2005b: 2). This concept has been discussed quite extensively by Rowling (1996) and elucidates the particular benefits of health promotion using the school environment strategically, and how it is superior to other public health strategies. The approach deliberately partners with parents, external agencies and the broader community (Hazell 2005b), and intentionally creates opportunities for professional development for school staff.

MindMatters was developed by an education and research consortium in 1997/1998 and was first piloted in 1998 and 1999 in twenty-four schools across Australia, specifically including rural and remote schools (Sheehan *et al.* 2002). This consortium primarily recognised that staff needed education in teaching for mental health as well as about mental health (Sheehan *et al.* 2002) if matters that were specifically identified as areas of concern were to be addressed. Examples of these were family issues, bullying and harassment, academic pressure, and drug use and depression. Further, as this was a health promotion project, it also included fostering supportive school environments, encouraging resilience and increasing the opportunities for development of self-esteem and social skills in young people (Sheehan *et al.* 2002).

Reportedly, this project is well based on the best evidence available (Hazell 2005b), including:

- that 'whole school' approaches are most effective for mental health promotion;
- prevention of harmful behaviours;
- risk and protective factors;
- effects of bullying;
- youth suicide research;
- mental health literacy among young people.

Stage 1: what is the specific intended purpose of the programme?

The broad aim of the MindMatters programme is to enhance the development of school environments so that young people feel safe, valued, engaged and purposeful (Ainley *et al.* 2006). The school environment has been determined as being crucial for social and emotional development in young people, and for their future ability to contribute purposefully in the workforce (Ainley *et al.* 2006). However, while the purpose of MindMatters is to promote wellbeing, it specifically aims to do this by creating a professional development programme for mental health promotion that is suitable for adoption in (all) secondary schools in Australia, as reported by the Commonwealth Department of Health and Aged Care (cited in Sheehan *et al.* 2002). The purpose of this undertaking is that schools become more aware of mental health issues, and foster the development of positive mental health.

Because of this chosen strategy, all students in government and independent secondary schools are targeted for mental health promotion. This is a large undertaking and undoubtedly a costly one. However, given the substantial evidence base for the value of this type of intervention, from a public health perspective it may prove to be judicious and well-spent. Herein the government demonstrates a valuing of health as important, which is supportive of article 24 in the United Nations Convention regarding rights of children to health. Certainly the cost of mental illness for Australia is high, being the third leading cause of disease burden, as reported by the National Mental Health Report (Department of Health and Ageing 2007). Despite individualised access to mental health services, this burden is not reducing but growing, and this justifies the substantial financial outlay on prevention, using different strategies to those already tried.

Following training, teachers implement a package of modules (eight in all) that cover a range of topics. Some titles are: 'Enhancing Resilience', 'Dealing with Bullying and Harassment', 'Understanding Mental Illness' and 'Working with Diversity for Wellbeing'; all modules are available in the 'Resources and Downloads' section of the MindMatters website (www.mindmatters.edu.au). Within the modules there are worksheets, activities, games and discussion points, all designed to further students' life skills, and the emergence of 'well rounded' confident individuals (Ainley *et al.* 2006).

As this programme is intended to create positive mental health in young people, it does not concentrate on any particular individual student or groups in its delivery. This is good human rights practice because it treats all students equally (UN General Assembly 1948), and makes the assumption that they can all benefit from the strategies. Further, it values the health of children as equal to that of adults (UN

General Assembly 1948), and aims to prevent ill health rather than delay intervention until poor health is detected.

However, it does not target children before secondary school-level education. This would indicate a belief that the years from 12 to 18 in a young person's life are the most important for this intervention, as indicated by Cummings (cited in Sheehan *et al.* 2002). There are conflicting viewpoints on this matter though, indicating, for example, the need for such programmes at a primary-school level (Short 1998), so that young people can develop positive mental health attitudes and resilience earlier in life (Wilkinson and Marmot 2003).

This intervention also does not provide maximum benefit to early school leavers, (before completion of year 12), potentially leaving lesser educated young people in society at higher risk. Unfortunately, this is possibly the group in which need of this intervention is highest, as indicated by Wilkinson and Marmot (2003) in their discussion of the social determinants of health, and is therefore a failing of this intervention from a human rights perspective. It could be considered to be discriminatory practice, as outlined in the Universal Declaration of Human Rights (UN General Assembly 1948) under article 25. There are possibly embedded beliefs evident around this failing of the intervention, as to the low economic value of 'school dropouts'. Excluding those who take up trades, as a group they would often be meagre contributors to society's net worth, so perhaps in the government's view they do not merit more directed social investment.

Stage 2: what are the ways and the extent to which the project may impact positively and negatively on health?

This project has been evaluated by a number of authors from the professional development perspective (Askell-Williams *et al.* 2005; Hazell 2005a), but there is a lack of a public health evaluation of the overall impact on students, probably because of the inherent difficulties of evaluating wellbeing, rather than emotional problems (Rowling *et al.* 2002). It is likely that longitudinal and qualitative studies will demonstrate the effectiveness of this intervention; however these are usually more costly and less likely to be conducted (Glasziou and Longbottom 1999). So public health has yet to adequately prove the effectiveness of this project, relying instead on subjective teacher experience (Hazell 2005b). This poses human rights questions, in that while the cost is high to run this project, the overall effectiveness may, ultimately, be low. This would then indicate that the funds might be more usefully employed elsewhere. Some schools indicate that students' knowledge, attitudes and behaviour improved (Askell-Williams *et al.* 2005), and their positive mental health attitudes and behaviour continued to improve past the teaching phase. This study however was conducted on a very small scale (three schools in the same state) and could not be claimed to be generalisable (Oliver and Peersman 2002).

The project could negatively impact students with specific mental health problems, through lack of recognition of their issues. This could occur because MindMatters' success is intended to be measured through wellbeing studies. If a young person feels well, does this mean they are? Are they more or less likely to experience mental illness? Martin (cited in Rowling *et al.* 2002) contends that this sole measure is likely to be adequate for most students, but may be problematic for those with specific undiagnosed illnesses.

However, there are many ways in which MindMatters can create benefit to health, and these are broader than mental health and long-lasting. Evidence indicates that when students are educated about negotiation skills, they are less likely to be violent to achieve their objective. This benefits women's health specifically in potentially reducing the occurrence of domestic violence (Victorian Health Promotion Foundation 2004). Also, when students identify they are stressed, they are more likely to seek assistance, reducing the levels of high blood pressure and heart disease in society (Butler 2004). Thirdly, when students are anxious they may employ positive strategies to come to a decision, rather than take up tobacco or alcohol consumption (Chapman 1993).

As these are some of the likely benefits of the MindMatters project, there is good reason to require all students to participate. Because human rights also imply responsibilities to society, it is arguable that students have a responsibility to maintain their health as well as they can (Wakefield 1997), and these skills may be crucial to their ability to do so.

Stage 3: what and whose rights are impacted positively and negatively by the programme?

This programme appears to be well targeted, aiming to instigate positive mental health behaviours and attitudes in young people. Schools are optimally placed to promote health when young people are developing mentally, and considering their attitudes to their environment (Short 1998). It is their right to health, not just the absence of illness, which is supported by this intervention.

There has not been demonstrated to be a better model for public mental health promotion in Australia. As an example of this, government talks about a youth mental health crisis as regards suicide, but currently prevention projects have not been effectively evaluated (Mitchell 2000). Conversely, a number of authors have reported on the benefits of 'health promoting schools' (Short 1998; Lister-Sharp *et al.* 1999; Bond *et al.* 2001; Stewart-Brown 2006).

Rowling (1996) is of particular interest, as she discusses how this concept can be used in Australian schools. Her work synthesises international experiences, and argues the reasons it can work here in even more beneficial ways. One of these is the common philosophy that she identifies in both health and education documents about outcomes for both sectors (Rowling 1996). Another is that the national government provides policy direction and financial support for both education and health. For equity of access this creates an excellent environment for promoting health, as it equally distributes resources across the country. It maximises the benefits of two government departments working together cooperatively.

It is possible, however, that over-inclusion has occurred in this project. As some children seem to develop resilience independently of the school system (Panter-Brick 2002), it is questionable whether it is necessary to enrol all students in it. Yet, for the development of a just society, which the values of the programme support, it may be beneficial for those who are more resilient to recognise that others are less so. As this programme aims to teach and model positive relationships between people, valuing differences related to diversity and resolving conflict (Sheehan *et al.* 2002), it is hard to suggest that such a programme would have negative consequences from this over-inclusion. In fact it is good human rights practice to create environments which emphasise the value of difference (Gearty 2006).

Under-inclusion is also evident, in that not all schools have sent staff to the professional development training, and this leaves 20 per cent of the student population of Australia unable to benefit from it (Hazell 2005b). Further, it was reported by the same evaluators that some rural and remote schools have not been able to access the training, for reasons related to school finances. Given that most services are difficult to access in these areas, it is most unfortunate that these schools have not been enabled to attend the training, as other reports evidence that they, in particular, have a greater benefit from the programme (Ainley *et al.* 2006). From a human rights perspective this is patently unjust, and discriminatory, when it seems to need only the funding of replacement teachers to facilitate access to the programme for these schools. The latest evaluation (ACER 2010) confirms that the programme is not in use in all schools, with 77 per cent of the schools in the sample reporting that they have used at least some aspect of MindMatters in the last three years. This figure is likely to be an overestimate of the actual percentage across all Australian schools, given the very low response rate reported for the survey.

Stage 4: does the programme necessitate the restriction of human rights?

The secondary school environment does not create extra restriction of behaviour, because the state already has legislated access to young people through the education system (Department of Education and Early Childhood Development 2007). It could be argued, though, that it is an unnecessary intrusion into the lives of students. All parents may not agree with its incorporation in the curriculum, although the programme aims to actively engage them as partners.

It could, further, be conceived that in some ways this intervention is a contravention of article 19 in the Universal Declaration of Human Rights (United Nations 1948) in that it does not allow students absolute freedom to think and speak freely. For example, the professional development training focuses, in part, on how to deal with bullying from a positive mental health perspective. This intentionally changes how students identified as 'bullies' interact with others.

On the other hand, it can be supported that article 1 in the Universal Declaration of Human Rights (United Nations 1948) requires that all people, students included, have a responsibility to treat others kindly and equally (Gearty 2006). This programme is therefore upholding a broad education of students in human rights, without specifically using that term. As it has long been noted that one human right is not held to be more important than others, it becomes a question of what is considered to be the greater good in the circumstances.

Lastly, it is also considered to be a human right that young people have access to quality education, as reported in article 28 in the Convention on the Rights of the Child. This education about fair practices in life is good human rights practice.

Stage 5: have the preconditions to restrict rights been met?

In discussing whether it is justified to restrict human rights to implement this programme, it is helpful to consider the Siracusa principles. They were devised by the United Nations in 1984 to examine justifications of limitations to human rights (ECOSOC 1984).

Of particular interest are four principles about human rights restrictions. First, the question is whether the restriction is lawful. As discussed earlier, the national government already has legal and educational access to students in secondary schools. Therefore, a new law has not been created to enable the conduct of this programme (Department of Education and Early Childhood Development 2007).

Secondly, the question is whether there is a legitimate objective of general interest. ECOSOC (1984) expresses this as responding to a 'pressing public or social need'. The then Health Minister was quite definitive about the need for effective health promotion. He reported that the child and adolescent component of the National Survey of Mental Health and Wellbeing revealed that 14 per cent of children and adolescents in Australia have mental health problems (Department of Health and Ageing 2000). This alarm led to the large-scale dissemination of this project, which before that point had only been trialed in twenty-four schools.

Next is the question of whether the restriction is necessary to achieve this objective. Apparently there are no other programmes that have proven effectiveness for mental health promotion (Mitchell 2000). While this is the case, or until this programme is proven ineffective (Short 1998; Bond et al. 2001), it could justify this limitation of human rights.

Lastly is the question of whether a less restrictive means is available for mental health promotion. This includes consideration of whether human rights restrictions are discriminatory. While the programme does not appear to be intentionally discriminatory, it makes assumptions that could be culturally discriminatory. For example, the term 'mental health' often translates poorly, or has no equivalent, in other languages (Barsh 1996). In relation to indigenous Australians, their understanding of such issues is commonly articulated as spiritual concerns and 'connection to land' (Armstrong 2002). This raises the question of whether mental health and human rights are concepts of Western society, which may not integrate with non-Western cultures (Sharma 2006).

This element does not mean that the programme is discriminatory, but would indicate that cultural considerations are vital to avoid discrimination (Eisenbruch et al. 2004). Otherwise, culturally and linguistically diverse groups, who already suffer poorer mental health and at significantly higher rates (Brough et al. 2003), will continue to be overrepresented, thereby creating a growing health inequity.

Stage 6: are health and other structures and services capable of effectively implementing the programme?

Given that this project was aimed to be run through secondary schools, with the assistance of local partner organisations, it was reasonably independent of other structures and services. It is interesting to note then that in places where there are less services (rural and remote areas), this project worked more effectively. In evaluation, it was noted quite strongly that much of the success had to do with school size and geographical location, and sometimes also community size (Ainley *et al.* 2006). Against trend, it became evident that the smaller the school and local community, the more powerful the intervention was. Sizeable metropolitan schools that exist in a resource-rich environment were less happy with the project results.

This indicates that more tailoring is necessary so that larger schools can equally benefit from the project. Perhaps stronger partnering is indicated, but also harder to achieve, in a less cohesive community. From a human rights perspective it is good practice to favour groups most at risk (Calma 2008), often identified as rural and remote, thereby reducing health discrimination and supporting the reduction of health inequities.

Stage 7: what system of monitoring, evaluation, accountability and redress exists?

MindMatters have published multiple reports on their website (www.mindmatters.edu.au) that are viewable by the general public. These have been conducted by research groups that are separate from the initial consortium that developed the project. Significantly though, there are no mechanisms for students to feed back their experience of the project, to a level other than the immediate classroom. Their selected comments have been recorded in the evaluations, but there are no other mechanisms by which they can contribute to the revision of this project. This demonstrates a lack of valuing of the students' experience and perspectives on mental health promotion, which is poor human rights practice. Young people can equally contribute to research involving them, and have a right to do so (Panter-Brick 2002).

Conclusion

MindMatters, through its implementation in secondary schools, has supported many human rights. It has utilised an accepted environment to promote mental health, using evidence to guide the project. However, for the MindMatters project to be considered good human rights practice, there are some areas for improvement. Discrimination is evident against early school leavers, rural and remote students and, potentially, mentally ill students. There are also concerns regarding language-appropriateness of the project with students from non-Western societies. MindMatters also needs to be careful about how it implements the lessening of freedoms of speech. Further, the project needs to consider how it will incorporate student participation, and improve the effectiveness of its implementation for larger schools.

11 The instrumental value of human rights in health

Brad Crammond

A human right to health was first proclaimed in the Constitution of the World Health Organization in 1946 and was reiterated in a different form – a right to a standard of living adequate for the health and wellbeing of himself and of his family – in the Universal Declaration of Human Rights in 1948. The right to health has since appeared in many forms in different human rights documents but its definitive statement appears as article 12 in the International Covenant on Economic, Social and Cultural Rights (UN General Assembly 1966a) and is worth repeating here:

1. The States Parties to the present Covenant recognize the right of everyone to the enjoyment of the highest attainable standard of physical and mental health.
2. The steps to be taken by the States Parties to the present Covenant to achieve the full realization of this right shall include those necessary for:
   (a) The provision for the reduction of the stillbirth-rate and of infant mortality and for the healthy development of the child;
   (b) The improvement of all aspects of environmental and industrial hygiene;
   (c) The prevention, treatment and control of epidemic, endemic, occupational and other diseases;
   (d) The creation of conditions which would assure to all medical service and medical attention in the event of sickness.

Article 12 represents the first serious attempt by the international community to define, in a human rights document, what countries must do if they are to fulfil the right to health. Thus, according to ICESCR it is the obligation of every government to progressively realise improvements in health generally and the indicators laid out in subarticle 2 specifically to the maximum of their available resources. These obligations are further strengthened and clarified in the Committee on Economic Social and Cultural Rights' *General Comment 14 on the Right to the Highest Attainable Standard of Health* (CESCR 2000) but the specifics of the minimum core obligations need not divert us here.

Each of the standards laid out in human rights documents show that, as a matter of human rights protection and fulfilment, governments must take seriously the health of the populations within their borders. If a government is neglecting public health, these statements of human rights principles are supposed to spur governments to change their ways. This chapter will consider whether human rights are conceptually able to play this role in the context of resource restrictions which are not themselves breaches of human rights.

As other chapters have discussed, the impetus for developing a *rights-based approach to health* was the global reaction to the spread of HIV/AIDS. In many countries health policies were eschewed for approaches which focused on quarantine or incarceration. In these cases it was possible to show that policies which violated human rights principles were also detrimental to health: policies of incarceration discouraged people from seeking HIV tests, which prevented health professionals from identifying those in need of health care or those who required education on how to prevent transmission to others (Mann *et al.* 1999). In extreme situations such as these, the value of human rights analyses to improve health policy-making is clear.

As treatment has become more widely available globally, the emphasis upon human rights as being the basis, or even an important component, of the response to HIV/AIDS has lessened (Gruskin *et al.* 2007). In keeping with this trend, the World Health Organization's Commission on Social Determinants of Health chose not to utilise human rights in its analysis of the relationship between social conditions and health. The following section will consider the debate around the role of human rights in the Commission's work and argue that human rights can be more useful than the Commission suggests.

Beyond the work of the Commission there are two areas in which human rights principles can be of significant instrumental value to health policy-making and programming. I will go on to examine the role of human rights in advocating for improvements to health services and social determinants. There have been some major successes in using human rights as the basis for advocacy, particularly in countries where protection of human rights is enshrined in law. I will then discuss the role of human rights principles in allocative decision-making processes. In these situations enumerated human rights are unable to provide a specific resolution and yet they can be used to construct a process which upholds human rights principles.

Social determinants of health

The recent Commission on the Social Determinants of Health (CSDH) examined the causes and extent of disparities in health between rich and poor worldwide. Set up in 2005 by the then Director-General of the World Health Organization, the CSDH was given 'the mission to collect and synthesize global evidence on the social determinants of health, assess their impact on health inequity, and make recommendations for action to address that inequity' (Venkatapuram *et al.* 2010: 4). Upon publication of the Commission's final report (CSDH 2008) Paul Hunt, recently retired as special rapporteur on the right to the highest attainable standard of health, described the Commission's failure to embrace a human rights approach as a 'series of missed opportunities' (Hunt 2009: 40). Hunt argues that the report of the CSDH is, in many ways, a human rights report, because the issues it canvases – equality and non-discrimination, poverty, access to basic shelter, food, education and health-related services – are also covered by the human rights documents. He further argues that the health and human rights discipline has matured greatly since its inception and now includes a suite of tools for implementation, including the use of indicators, benchmarks, impact assessments, budgetary analysis and different types of accountability (Hunt 2009).

In their defence of the CSDH report Venkatapuram, Bell and Marmot (the Chair of the CSDH) argue that human rights may play an instrumental role in obtaining the goods and services required to resolve the problems identified with epidemiology, but that they add no explanatory power to a health problem (Venkatapuram *et al.* 2010). That is, when epidemiology or other research disciplines identify health needs, the role of human rights is in providing grounds for advocacy, but does not provide any additional assistance in identifying needs. To illustrate this claim, Venkatapuram *et al.* consider Paul Farmer's (2008) example of a Malawian hospital where maternal mortality is low by in-country standards but very high by global standards. Within the hospital, shortages of medical supplies contribute to the maternal mortality rate, particularly shortages of sutures, sterile drapes and anaesthesia. If the failure to provide sutures is both a cause of a poor health outcome and also a human rights violation, what role can human rights play with respect to a cause which is not itself a breach of a listed human right? To put it another way, how can or should human rights law deal with causes of human rights violations which are not violations in and of themselves? There is no enumerated human right to sutures, though the lack of sutures might in this context violate the broader right to health.

Venkatapuram *et al.* (2010) consider three paths that a human rights proponent might take in responding to the lack of a right to sutures. Path 1 would attempt to read a right to sutures into existing human rights provisions. Path 2 would derive general principles from human rights law and seek to demonstrate that the failure to provide sutures violates one of these general principles. Path 3 would 'back away from the arena of human rights law and would instead attempt to bridge the analysis of the causes and distribution of ill health and mortality on the ground with ethical reasoning about social justice' (Venkatapuram *et al.* 2010: 10). The Commission chose path 3 because ultimately 'members of the Commission were not convinced that explicit consideration of the legal human right to health changed their final causal analysis' (Venkatapuram *et al.* 2010: 7).

It is uncontroversial that in many respects human rights action is dependent upon the social sciences for its content. The work of a broad range of groups, from clinicians to anthropologists to journalists, has been instrumental in bringing to public notice human rights abuses. The first path suggested by Venkatapuram *et al.* is a great simplification of this relationship. According to this path, the specific causes of any rights violation (in this case a lack of sutures) would themselves be treated as human rights. The consequences of such an approach to human rights scholarship would be dire, robbing human rights of any separate or distinctive conceptual content. Consequently it is not a position supported by human rights proponents. Instead, the preferred way to conceive of the relationship between scientific evidence and human rights is to see evidence as part of a supportive process helping to elucidate what compliance with human rights requires in different settings. Thus rather than treating the lack of sutures as requiring a human right to sutures, the lack can be seen as an example of how the right to health is being violated in this context. Providing sutures therefore becomes an element of fulfilling the right to health and not a standalone right.

Using scientific evidence to fill out the content of human rights in this way is not considered as an option by Venkatapuram *et al*. Instead, they question the instrumental value of human rights at all on the basis that in some countries the promotion of human rights is more controversial than is the promotion of health. Though it is true that in some countries there is well-documented resistance to the use of human rights in health programmes, these countries certainly represent a minority of countries in the world. In the great majority of countries human rights may be regularly violated but none argue that human rights are irrelevant or inappropriate standards. The strength of human rights is even greater in the international system where the United Nations has declared that human rights form the basis of all programmes and policies, where the World Health Organization proclaims health to be a human right and where most secular aid agencies are motivated by the aim of improving human rights enjoyment. When dealing with such institutions, recourse to human rights principles is unlikely to ever be counter-productive. Venkatapuram *et al*. (2010) therefore base their rejection of the instrumental value of human rights on the opposition of only a small group of countries and ignore the many other countries and agencies which take claims of human rights violations very seriously.

Path 2, distilling human rights principles from the treaties and using these principles as analytical tools, is rightly identified as placing the cart before the horse, although it is often forgotten that human rights principles represent only one of many different conceptions of social justice. Other theories, like the capabilities approach propounded (1999, 2009) by Amartya Sen (one of the members of the CSDH), or the liberal egalitarianism of John Rawls (1971), provide more comprehensive accounts of what justice requires than do human rights. In fact, human rights are themselves merely the outcomes of a theory of democratic liberalism. Unlike the other theories, human rights have been instantiated as international and national law, but in the negotiation required to achieve this feat have ceased to accurately represent any particular theory of social justice. Thus many human rights proponents have proven unable to posit a philosophical basis for all the human rights listed in the many human rights treaties (Freeman 1994; Shestack 1998). Since ethical reasoning preceded and is responsible for human rights legislation, Venkatapuram *et al*. (2010) argue that it is better to rely directly on this reasoning.

Consequently, the CSDH chose to follow the third path which is to rely on ethical reasoning directly rather than foreground human rights. In situations where questions of health distribution across the income spectrum or the causes of health failures are not themselves human rights, recourse to ethical reasoning will always provide greater nuance and subtlety than is possible from a human rights analysis. At the same time, however, such ethical reasoning and the training required to perform it is not naturally incorporated into health. A public health practitioner schooled in epidemiology and not lucky enough to have a personal friendship with Amartya Sen (as is the case with Michael Marmot) will find it substantially easier to derive a basic understanding of human rights as they apply to her work than she will to learn the many complexities of social justice theory. Furthermore, their arguments are likely to be more easily comprehensible to others (including politicians) who are similarly unfamiliar with detailed ethical reasoning. In many respects the weaknesses described by Venkatapuram *et al.* (2010) may also be considered strengths of the human rights system. Where they see simplicity as a shortcoming, in a context where most people working in health have only the most limited exposure to any theories of justice, the simplicity provided by human rights makes it manageable. If one was to choose between complex ethical reasoning and human rights, human rights would always be second best. But as the only available form of ethical reasoning human rights undoubtedly direct attention to some important aspects of justice and their use is unlikely to make health policy less just.

The more important point here, though, is a failure on the part of the CSDH to recognise the contingent nature of the current consensus on health promotion. Unlike human rights, ethical precepts supporting international action to promote health, particularly in developing countries, are not enshrined in international law. They do not form the basis of institutional practices and they do not have the stated support of every nation. It was not so long ago that the health of populations in developing countries was of concern to Europe only by virtue of its capacity to frustrate colonialism. It seems short-sighted to reject the enormous volume of negotiation and advocacy which has led to the acceptance of human rights in favour of the relatively recently established non-controversial nature of health promotion.

Paul Hunt is right to say that the Commission's work is a missed opportunity for health and human rights. Though it is possible, as the CSDH shows, to combine health and justice without relying upon human rights, doing so needlessly discards important principles. Human rights remain internationally recognised and accepted, unlike the alternative ethical analyses proposed by the CSDH.

Choosing between health programmes and between disadvantaged populations

Rights-based approaches to health seek to shift public health decision-making so that it is more aware of the rights of disadvantaged populations and more respectful of human rights generally. It is clear to many human rights proponents, however, that the list of rights enumerated in the treaties does not provide a sufficient basis upon which to construct a nationwide health system. There are, for example, specific resource allocation decisions to be made between competing priorities for treatment within and between disadvantaged populations for which one can obtain little direct guidance from human rights principles. In these cases writers like Norman Daniels (2008) and Jennifer Ruger (2010) have recommended procedural approaches which are grounded in human rights principles like equality and non-discrimination as a way of making decisions which are consistent with human rights.

The limits of human rights decision-making

There are two types of decisions which are regularly made within a functioning health system: choosing between different interventions to treat a particular illness and choosing between interventions to be applied in different populations. Often the two decisions will overlap.

Let us take as an example a choice between addressing cardiovascular disease in rural and remote indigenous Australian populations, and providing sexual and reproductive health services to female refugees. Here the two types of decision overlap – first the decision-maker must choose between the best way to treat each condition and then choose between which population is most deserving (or the sequence may take place in the reverse order).

Australia's indigenous population has rates of cardiovascular disease (CVD) significantly higher than the non-indigenous population (Wang and Hoy 2005). Many possible public health responses are available. At an individual clinical level, the patient may have high blood pressure and cholesterol levels which can be treated with pharmaceuticals. Choosing to subsidise these medicines, as the government does in Australia, is a public health response to CVD and one which is respectful of human rights – providing medicine at a lower cost does not violate any human rights. Still at an individual level but looking a little more broadly, a health department could introduce a policy to provide education about the importance of diet and exercise to anyone who presents in hospital with CVD, with the aim of reducing the impact of those two factors which are closely associated with CVD. This second response does not violate any human rights, instead promoting freedom of expression (which includes the right to receive information) (ICCPR, article 19.2) along with the right to health. Moving to a community level, the health department could instigate a policy that high-risk groups for CVD should be targeted and provided with education about the importance of good diet and sufficient exercise. This approach may reduce the number of people presenting to hospital, preventing the disease rather than managing it once it has already developed. This approach may even be more effective than the first two mentioned, but it is equal in not placing any burden on human rights. At a final community level, the health department may recognise that high stress levels contribute to CVD when people have low capability to cope with that stress and that indigenous people as a group have lower capabilities to cope with stress owing to their history of social disruption, poverty and substandard education (Baum 1998). The best way to address these problems could be responses not traditionally associated with public health, like improving education standards generally (not just about CVD) and providing assistance in reshaping social structures so that indigenous people have more supportive and less stressful communities. Implemented in a sensitive and respectful way, this final approach will also be consistent with human rights standards. The most effective response may in fact be a combination of all four. The final approach, though providing the greatest fulfilment of the greatest number of human rights, provides little immediate assistance to those already suffering from CVD; the third approach could help with prevention but may reinforce stereotypes about at-risk populations if not implemented sensitively; the first and second approaches provide treatment but do little in the way of prevention for those who are at risk.

It is, therefore, not clear from a human rights analysis which policy should be chosen by the health department. Even when modelling of the likely reductions in ill health and economic cost are factored in it will not be clear, on a human rights basis, which policy is the best (though it may be clear on an economic basis which has the advantage of reducing all of human experience to a single indicator). A more extensive range of options could be presented for refugee women, with the same problem of resolution.

As between the two populations, human rights principles generally direct attention toward the most vulnerable in society. The focus on the disadvantaged is most clearly laid out in the Committee on Economic Social and Cultural Rights' General Comment 3 on the Nature of States Parties Obligations. It states that 'even in times of severe resource constraint ... the vulnerable members of society can and indeed must be protected by the adoption of relatively low-cost targeted programmes' (CESCR 1990: para 12). This is the first reference to a general vulnerability in which multiple rights may be unfulfilled and which does not reference a specific political or other characteristic. According to this comment, the people who are most vulnerable (though to what is unspecified) are the first subjects of economic, social and cultural rights: only when their basic needs are met should states consider increasing the rights enjoyment of other more powerful (or at least less vulnerable) groups. Focusing on the groups with the lowest human rights enjoyment first should still be the priority in situations of resource non-scarcity since it is logical that, as resources increase, services should be prioritised first to the most vulnerable, then the next most vulnerable and so on. That human rights focus on the most vulnerable members of society has now become a commonplace statement in General Comments. All of the treaty bodies have mentioned vulnerability as a prioritising factor, though few of the references are as comprehensive as that made by CESCR in General Comment 3. It is not possible, however, from these statements to choose clearly between refugee women and indigenous populations as being the most vulnerable or disadvantaged.

Accountability for Reasonableness

In recognition of the limitations of decision-making based on human rights, Norman Daniels has developed a procedural approach for all those decisions which human rights cannot clearly answer, called Accountability for Reasonableness (Daniels 2008; Gruskin and Daniels 2008). Borrowing from democratic theory he argues that a fair procedure is the only way to resolve resource allocation decisions where there is more than one option which is consistent with human rights, as in the example provided above. This procedure has some important limitations, however, which illustrate the difficulties in using human rights to make fine-grained decisions about health policy. This section will outline Daniels' theory before canvassing some of the criticisms.

Accountability for Reasonableness was originally presented as a way of resolving allocation decisions which could not be determined by recourse to a theory of health justice alone. Daniels's account of health justice is based upon John Rawls's account of social justice presented in the seminal political philosophical work

A Theory of Justice (Rawls 1971). In his most recent presentation of this account Daniels argues that health should be protected because it is a prerequisite for normal functioning in society (Daniels 2008). Though this account differs somewhat in its emphasis on particular rights and liberties, there is sufficient agreement that it has also been presented as being relevant to decision-making based on human rights principles (Gruskin and Daniels 2008).

Thus when a decision is to be made between, for example, cardiovascular disease prevention in indigenous groups and providing reproductive services to refugees, the way to resolve the problem is through an open decision-making process with input from relevant groups and individuals. According to Gruskin and Daniels (2008), there are four essential conditions for this process:

1 Publicity condition: decisions that establish priorities in meeting health needs and their rationales must be publicly accessible.
2 Relevance condition: the rationales for priority-setting decisions should aim to provide a reasonable explanation of why the priorities selected were determined to be the best approach. Specifically, a rationale is reasonable if it appeals to evidence, reasons, and principles accepted as relevant by fair-minded people. Closely linked to this condition is the inclusion of a broad range of stakeholders in decision-making.
3 Revision and appeals condition: there must be mechanisms for challenge and dispute and, more broadly, opportunities for revision and improvement of policies in light of new evidence or arguments.
4 Regulative condition: there must be public regulation of the process to ensure that conditions 1, 2 and 3 are met. (Gruskin and Daniels 2008)

The first, third and fourth elements are staples of participatory decision-making. The publicity condition is essential if the wider population is to be involved in the decisions that governments and bureaucracies make. Without transparency in what and how decisions are made, any participation from those other than the specific decision-makers will be uninformed and unlikely to be relevant. The revision and appeals condition ensures that decisions can be changed once their practical effect is known so that people are not burdened by the unintended consequences of otherwise fairly made decisions. Again this is essential if members of the wider population, who will have the most intimate knowledge of how policies affect them, are to achieve the best possible outcome. Finally the regulative condition provides accountability of decision-making by placing control of the process in the hands of the populace rather than the decision-maker.

It is the second element, the relevance condition, which is the primary innovation of Daniels's approach. The purpose of the relevance condition is to ensure that the reasons for making decisions between groups are based upon measures which are consistent with the liberal desire for rationality and are therefore as objective as possible. In our example appropriate principles would be the potential health benefit of each intervention, the current suffering experienced by each population or the extent of governmental responsibility for the health problems. It would be inappropriate, on the other hand, to rely on principles such as racist doctrines regarding the superiority of one race over another, sexist beliefs regarding the greater importance of men over women or nationalistic ideas which prioritise white Australians over 'undeserving foreigners'.

Once inappropriate principles are excluded, there remains more than one rational approach to the decision-making. Refugee advocacy groups could legitimately and rationally argue that refugee women have suffered in their country of origin and potentially in Australia as well if they were subject to immigration detention. On this basis, apart from their obvious health needs, as a matter of not further compounding their human rights abuses, the women should be entitled to appropriate care. Indigenous advocacy groups could just as legitimately and rationally argue that indigenous people have suffered greatly at the hands of settlers and that cardiovascular disease is merely the latest manifestation of a white system which discriminates against the indigenous. Thus, having violated their rights to the enjoyment of their culture (ICESCR, article 15), and their right to self-determination (ICESCR, article 1; ICCPR, article 1), governments have a responsibility to now take action to reduce heart disease in indigenous communities. In each case arguments will satisfy the relevance condition and yet a decision-maker is no closer to being able to decide between interventions for the two groups, or which intervention within the group is most appropriate.

Gruskin and Daniels (2008) concede that in many resource allocation decisions there will be 'winners and losers'. Accordingly, if the hypothetical decision-maker in this example was to choose to fund the reproductive services on the grounds put forward by the advocates, the decision will satisfy the requirements of Accountability for Reasonableness (provided the other conditions are met). It is obviously not ideal that only one service is provided, but where there are insufficient resources to fund all worthy programmes, provided that decisions are made on relevant criteria, the decision is to be held as being consistent with human rights. Of course, in practice, it might be possible to fund both projects at lower levels or to shift resources from health services provided to less vulnerable groups.

The primary criticism of this process for decision-making is that it fails to provide any more guidance than the human rights principles on their own (Rid 2009). The relevance condition requires that rationale be based upon 'principles accepted as relevant by fair-minded people' and the stipulation of 'fair-minded' suggests that a majority decision is not what is envisaged. Instead it suggests that people who already accept human rights as important guiding principles make decisions on those principles. But if, as Daniels argues, those principles are not determinative there appears to be a gap in terms of what principles or other ideas they are to use to decide the issue. That is, human rights are not determinative and yet they form the basis of the principles upon which fair-minded people are to rely. Similarly, the sorts of reasons which are incompatible with the relevance condition are also incompatible with human rights. Reasoning based on racism, sexism or other forms of discrimination, for example, falls foul both of the relevance condition and the human rights prohibition on discrimination. This circularity goes to the heart of efforts to combine substantive and procedural approaches to justice.

Consider the potential outcomes of a decision-making process. Any decision made utilising this process must be considered invalid if it violates human rights in some way. This is necessary because the substantive principles of human rights take precedence over the procedural aspect (which is only invoked when the substantive principles fail to provide a specific answer). At a high level of generality decisions to allocate significant resources to defence rather than to health may violate the right to health, though relevant and rational arguments can be made about the importance of defence to national security and individual rights to personal security (ICCPR, article 9). Outcomes of the process must, therefore, fall within a boundary of outcomes consistent with human rights. The process itself does not therefore make a decision consistent with human rights; rather it merely provides a justifiable way of deciding between alternatives which have already been deemed consistent. This proviso weakens the model to merely being a filter over various choices rather than a free-standing aid to human rights-consistent decision-making.

The use of human rights principles in decision-making in health can clearly identify areas which are and which are not consistent with human rights. Simply relying on the human rights treaties, however, does not provide guidance as to how decisions should be made between interventions which equally promote human rights, or between populations equally deserving of assistance. A procedural approach can assist decision-makers in selecting and justifying the selection of one intervention over another, but it cannot provide a perfect approach to problems of resource allocation.

Conclusion

Human rights, as enshrined in the many international treaties, now form part of the legal obligations that states owe the people within their control. In the arena of health, human rights direct attention towards populations which are the most disadvantaged but fail to provide clear answers to how resources should be allocated within and between different populations. They do not provide any additional analytical strength to the epidemiological evidence regarding the social determinants of health and they likewise fail to provide clear answers to how best to choose between competing interventions.

This is not to say, however, that human rights principles are irrelevant to health, rather that claims to their relevance must be circumscribed. To the extent that human rights have international clout they can and should be used to further the cause of improving health worldwide – in many cases, though, the imperative of improving population health has more resonance with policy-makers than do human rights concerns. This situation may not reflect well upon the international community but any claims to the instrumental value of human rights must be cognisant of its persistent association for some with accusations of Western imperialism (Donnelly 1999). Furthermore, the fundamental role of human rights work is to relieve the absolute deprivation in the world which is a sufficiently noble cause without also claiming that human rights are relevant to every health policy decision, especially those in the industrialised world.

Human rights are indescribably important to millions across the globe but this importance is only diluted by over-reaching claims of their usefulness.

Success or failure

How useful are rights-based approaches in public health?

WHO (2002a) makes a strong statement about the value of human rights work in health, and that human rights approaches provide a lever for seeking actions that protect and promote public health and provide important tools for tackling health inequity. Many examples of successful use of rights-based approaches can be found, and earlier chapters have already introduced some of these. WHO (2002a) posed the question: 'what is the value-added of human rights in public health?' Their answer to this question was set out as eleven different elements. In the first part of this final chapter, these eleven elements are used as a framework against which to summarise the evidence on what has been achieved over the past twenty or so years in terms of the usefulness of RBAs in public health.

Human rights may benefit work in the area of public health by providing explicit recognition of highest attainable standard of health as a 'human right' (as opposed to a good or commodity with a charitable construct)

Earlier chapters noted the link between many human rights, particularly economic and social rights, and the social determinants of health, it is thus appropriate to regard the achievement of human rights in itself as a social determinant of health. Work towards supporting all human rights directly contributes to supporting the right to health through support for the social determinants of health. Explicit recognition of a foundation for public health policy and practice in the realisation of human rights provides a powerful mandate, ultimately backed by international treaties and conventions with legal status, a value-based alternative to views of health as a commodity to be bought and sold in the marketplace, and a move away from argumentation for public health action based on paternalistic concepts of charity. Human rights-based approaches are highly congruent with empowerment-based approaches now regarded as the foundation of effective health promotion, and of interactions between health professionals and their clients in many fields of practice. As Chapter 5 discussed, rights-based approaches support empowerment, reinforce health promotion and capacity building, are supportive of strengths-based (as opposed to deficits-focused) models and can contribute to reducing dependency. Examples are provided in Pepin *et al.* (2010), and Ife (2008) on rights-based practice in social work. Finally, Cook *et al.* (2003) provide a wealth of examples in reproductive and sexual health at the individual care level, and Coulter and Collins (2011) discuss how to achieve shared decision-making in clinical practice, so that clinicians and patients work together to select tests, treatments, management or support packages based on clinical evidence and the patient's informed preferences.

Human rights may benefit work in the area of public health by providing a tool to enhance health outcomes by using a human rights approach to designing, implementing and evaluating health policies and programmes

The second element in WHO's answer on the value added by human rights to public health has been evidenced throughout the second half of the book. Chapter 5 above considered a number of different RBAs used in design of policies and programmes. Some of these were explicitly linked to health policies and programmes, others were linked to closely related areas, particularly development planning/programming, human rights education and capacity building both individual and community-based. The last twenty years have seen considerable growth in the development and use of these approaches and, where they have been evaluated, they have, in the main, showed positive results in terms of health-related outcomes.

To give a brief recap of these, first of all in terms of the field of development there has been UNICEF's human rights-based approach to programming (Jonsson 2003). Silva (2003) discusses the common understanding achieved among the different UN agencies working in the field, while Nyamu-Musembi and Cornwall's review (2004) presents a critical perspective on the view of international development agencies about rights-based approaches, and identifies the need to achieve a positive transformation of power relations among the various development actors. Bakker *et al.* (2009) review the application of the Health Rights of Women Assessment Instrument (Aims for Human Rights 2008). They report that it is effective in that its application and the consequent demonstration of where existing or intending policies did not comply with human rights obligations of the government led to change in policies.

In terms of particular topics, HIV/AIDS has been a particularly significant area of focus, not without some debate about whether there are differences in different parts of the globe in how this should play out, and of value of human rights approaches in this context (e.g. De Cock *et al.* 2002). A second important area is in terms of access to services. Chapters 3 and 4 illustrated how rights-based approaches have improved access to services in many countries. A third important area is access to pharmaceuticals. Internationally, there has been a lot of successful work supporting the availability of essential medicines at low or no cost, for example Brazil's work in championing improved access to antiretrovirals (Galvão 2005; Nunn *et al.* 2009) and its collaboration with other countries such as Cuba (Lage 2011), and also the success of multiple countries reviewed in Hogerzeil *et al.* (2006) in using litigation to secure access to essential medicines for individuals or groups.

In terms of basic education on rights, Chapter 5 presented the example of a UK-based programme, Active Learning for Active Citizenship or ALAC, that worked with a variety of different disadvantaged groups that commonly experience discrimination, showing how ALAC was able to achieve effective outcomes for both individuals and groups in a wide range of different settings (Annette and Mayo 2010). Looking more internationally, WHO has produced two rights cartoon books in a variety of different languages to support education on rights, the first on the right to health (WHO 2002b) and the second on HIV/AIDS (WHO 2003a; updated in 2010).

Chopra and Ford (2005) discuss a human rights approach to health promotion, based on UNICEF's approach (Jonsson 2003). In their approach the emphasis is on the characteristics of a community's organisations and institutions rather than the content of the message. Sharing of experience and a strong learning process among a partnership drawing from both partners, state actors and civil society, helps scaling up to occur. This process must be planned strategically, and involve developing a common vision, being explicit about roles and responsibility and facilitating communication channels for the most vulnerable. They find that a human rights-based approach can facilitate such an approach. They conclude, however, that this necessitates health development agencies pursuing overtly political agendas.

In term of the use of rights-based approaches in design and evaluation, the detailed example considered in Chapter 5 was that of CARE International, one of the largest internationally operating agencies, who have not only developed a rights-based approach to their work but also evaluated this, both through a specific evaluation across sixteen different projects (Picard 2005), and through other publications (Igras *et al.* 2004; Sarelin 2007; Frisancho and Goulden 2008; Rand and Watson 2008). Looking at other literature, rights-based responses to HIV and drug use have had good outcomes where they have been implemented (Jürgens *et al.* 2010). Hargreaves *et al.* (2011), describe inter-sectoral collaboration around the Intervention with Microfinance for AIDS and Gender Equity (IMAGE) in South Africa. IMAGE combined an established microfinance programme with gender and HIV/AIDS training, and activities to support community mobilisation. They discuss expanding the scale of intervention delivery following a trial and exploring models for long-term sustainable delivery, in the context of the recognition of IMAGE as a successful rights-based intervention.

In contrast, Martinez and Phillips (2008), in an interview-based study of sexual health education in secondary schools, identify tensions resulting from a biomedical, risk-focused application of the 'Ontario Health and Physical Education' curriculum. Even though the health sector attempted to promote a rights-based approach to sexual and reproductive health, the study's findings indicated that inequities due to gender, race/ethnicity and sexuality and their intersections were reinforced rather than challenged. They argue that ensuring that teaching was consistent with the principles and practices set out in the guidelines for sexual health education formulated by Health Canada (2003, updated in 2008) would help in reducing discrimination. Martinez and Phillips's findings prompt the need for caution: rights-based approaches do not automatically lead to positive results; there may be failures in implementation, such as insufficient training or education, so that positive results are not achieved.

Finally in relation to this element in WHO's list of the value added of human rights to public health, there is the seven-stage method for human rights analysis of policies or programmes, originating in the work of Gostin and Mann (1994), discussed in Chapter 6. This is illustrated in application in four contrasting examples in Australia, Austria, India and South Africa in Chapters 7 to 10 and, as Chapter 6 discussed, has been used in other cases as well.

Human rights may benefit work in the area of public health by providing an 'empowering' strategy for health which includes vulnerable and marginalised groups engaged as meaningful and active participants

This third element in WHO's answer about the value added by human rights has already been touched on in the discussion of the second element above. Two of the examples considered in Chapter 5, CARE International and ALAC, provide detailed examples of the empowerment consequent on the use of rights-based approaches and how this enabled a much wider inclusion of diverse vulnerable, marginalised and disadvantaged groups. It is important to note however three shared findings from their evaluation: first, the question of allowing sufficient time for the work to take place; second, caution about the feasibility of long-term sustainability without outside facilitation or support; and third, the necessity for working with a wide range of stakeholders, both rights-holders and duty-bearers, with careful attention to analysis of power relations in the context concerned.

Here empowerment can be understood as 'the process of increasing capacity of individuals or groups to make choices and to transform those choices into desired actions and outcomes' (Alsop 2004: 120). Evidence on importance of empowerment for health outcomes comes from the review conducted by Wallerstein (2006) which demonstrates that: empowering initiatives lead to improved health outcomes (both directly and indirectly); participation alone is insufficient without capacity building; successful empowering interventions must be created or adapted to local contexts, for example gender and culture appropriateness. Empowerment is closely connected to the notion of autonomy, and Marmot summarises the importance of autonomy as follows: 'Autonomy – how much control you have over your life – and the opportunities you have for full social engagement and participation are crucial for health, well-being and longevity' (Marmot 2004: 2). In the context of rights-based approaches and empowerment specifically, strong evidence for this element is also provided in a variety of recent studies and reviews (Kapoor 2007; de Vos et al. 2009; Hopkins 2011; Wearing 2011; Bajaj 2012). Finally, Black Sash (2011) report on their work in South Africa, using RBAs to support stakeholder and community engagement in health policy formulation.

Human rights may benefit work in the area of public health by providing a useful framework, vocabulary and form of guidance to identify, analyse and respond to the underlying determinants of health

Elsewhere in the book, the considerable overlap between human rights, particularly economic, social and cultural rights, and the social determinants of health has been noted. Thus a human rights framework is of direct relevance to addressing the underlying determinants of health, and rights-based approaches play a key role. Work on poverty, equity and human rights needs to be closely linked, as Braveman and Gruskin (2003a) demonstrate in their paper which explores the concepts of poverty, equity, and human rights in relation to health and to each other, demonstrating that they are closely linked conceptually and operationally, and that each provides valuable, unique guidance for health institutions' work. Equity and human rights perspectives can contribute to health institutions' efforts to tackle poverty and health, and focusing on poverty is essential to operationalising those commitments. The work of CARE International, discussed in Chapter 5, provides one good example; their rights-based framework has served them well in their work which is aimed at addressing poverty, one of the major underlying determinants of health.

A further example of the potential is given in Mandel's (2006) paper for the New Economics Foundation (see case study). In terms of work on HIV/AIDS, Mann and Tarantola (1998: 5) identify four phases in the history of the response to HIV/AIDS. The transition from the third phase in which HIV/AIDS was seen as a societally contextualised behavioural issue to the fourth phase in which HIV/AIDS was seen as a human rights-linked challenge emerged from the recognition of the important roles of social marginalisation, stigmatisation and discrimination in vulnerability to HIV/AIDS, and the recognition that a form of analysis focused on the societal basis of vulnerability was required. The focus on social determinants of health within human rights provided a useful framework, vocabulary and guidance.

Human rights may benefit work in the area of public health by providing a standard against which to assess the performance of governments in health

The right to health has provided a basis for assessments of government performance in health. As discussed in Chapter 2, General Comment 14 (CESCR 2000) sets out standards in relation to the right to health and also expounds a set of core obligations (paragraphs 43 and 44). In terms of specific topics, HIV/AIDS and access to medicines provide examples of where more specific elaborations have been given (World Health Assembly 2000; Commission on Human Rights 2001). As mentioned in Chapter 6, the People's Health Movement, building on the work of Health Rights of Women Assessment Instrument (HeRWAI, see Aim for Human Rights 2008), has produced a guide to the assessment of the right to health and health care at the country level (PHM 2006). Similarly Hunt and MacNaughton (2006) provide an approach to assessing achievements in relation to the highest attainable standard of health. Backman *et al.* (2008) provide an assessment of 194 countries' achievements in relation to health systems and the right to health: using a set of seventy-two indicators drawing on globally available data. Lecomte and Mercier (2008) discuss how the WHO atlas on global resources for persons with intellectual disabilities and the international human rights instruments can form two parts of a holistic approach in regards to state-provided services to persons with intellectual disabilities and their families.

Case study: A human rights approach to debt relief

Aim: promote a concept of debt sustainability which puts rights and basic wellbeing of people first and those of the creditors second.

Starting point: the amount of revenue that a government can be expected to raise without increasing poverty or compromising future development. This means:

- not taxing people who already have less income than they need for basic rights;
- protecting government spending needed to meet basic human development needs.

Using data for 136 countries, Mandel calculates how much debt cancellation each country would need to reduce its debt to a sustainable level, and concludes that, on human rights grounds:

- between fifty-one and fifty-four countries need complete cancellation of their debts
- between thirty-two and fifty-three countries need partial cancellation.

In order to stop the drain on government budgets from debt servicing (which is one of the factors which prevents their meeting the basic needs of their populations), substantial debt cancellation is urgently needed.

A further implication is that none of the countries requiring debt cancellation can afford to take on more debt, though that is what has happened in the past. Yet they all need more resources, beyond the relief which could be provided by debt cancellation, if they are to meet the Millennium Development Goals and reduce poverty. There therefore needs to be a substantial increase in grant aid in addition to the debt cancellation proposed.

(Summarised from Mandel 2006)

Human rights may benefit work in the area of public health by providing enhanced governmental accountability for health

Chapters 2, 3 and 4 of this book have focused on the different human rights systems for monitoring and accountability at global, regional and national level, emphasising the variety in arrangements by which these systems can hold duty-bearers to account for rights violations and/or for lack of protection, promotion and fulfilment of human rights. The discussions have emphasised that examples can be found of where such systems have been instrumental in bringing about positive change, but positive change is by no means guaranteed. Some examples exist of governments responding, but also of them not responding. As has been demonstrated, possibilities of recourse to the legal system vary by country, but as has also been stressed, there are many possibilities and routes for change through advocacy in addition to use of the legal system, as Chapter 1 discussed.

There are also ongoing debates about whether there are strong cases to be made for proposing additional legislation in countries based on various treaties. Ingleby *et al.* (2008), for example, argue that there is a strong case to be made for proposing additional legislation in Australia based on the Convention on Rights of the Child to ban certain food advertisements on television.

Human rights may benefit work in the area of public health by providing a powerful authoritative basis for advocacy and cooperation with governments; international organisations; international financial institutions; and in the building of partnerships with relevant actors of civil society

As discussed in Chapter 3, Cabal *et al.* (2003) describe the work of the Center for Reproductive Rights in Latin America, and illustrate how international human rights litigation can help raise awareness of reproductive rights at national and international levels and lead to important legal and policy/practice change. Sanchez Fuentes *et al.* (2008) also demonstrated the effectiveness of rights-based argumentation in achieving the decriminalisation of abortion in Mexico City.

Examples of this work and its successes have been covered in detail in Chapter 5. Experience from two of the examples considered there, CARE International and ALAC, demonstrate that careful judgement is needed about whether to use the language of rights explicitly or not. Similar conclusions are reached in Berman (2008). Use of human rights approaches in the field of harm reduction is explored by Fox (2005), Fry *et al.* (2005) and Jacobson and Bannerjee (2005). Jacobson and Bannerjee (2005) consider how tobacco control strategies can use human rights framing in voluntary non-smoking strategies to their advantage, and Fox (2005) examines how public health needs to frame its efforts to counter the tobacco industry's use of 'rights argumentation' to position itself as the protector of individual rights. In the field of harm reduction, Fry *et al.* (2005) and Keane (2003) both offer distinctive critiques of the role of human rights approaches in harm reduction. Finally, in relation to specific population groups, Morgan and David (2002) discuss the usefulness of human rights principles for ageing advocacy and public education efforts.

Human rights may benefit work in the area of public health by providing existing international mechanisms to monitor the realisation of health as a human right

The international human rights system, through Universal Periodic Review, as well as the work of the treaty monitoring bodies and the work of the special rapporteurs, provides ample opportunity to monitor the realisation of health as a human right, with or without the assistance of various monitoring tools discussed above. It is vital however that focus is kept on examining the change that occurs over time, i.e. progress or not. This has led many people to call for explicit use of indicators and Backman *et al.* (2008) have taken up this challenge using globally processed data for 194 countries on seventy-two different indicators. There is also considerable debate over the value and difficulties associated with such approaches, see for example Felner (2009). As was noted above, examples exist of governments responding positively to the identification of problems and lack of progress, but also of them not responding.

Human rights may benefit work in the area of public health by providing accepted international norms and standards (e.g. definitions of concepts and population groups)

Chapters 1 and 2 earlier emphasised how the UN human rights systems are progressively being developed through key mechanisms including new treaties/conventions/protocols focused on particular groups and 'General Comments' issued by monitoring committees that help elaborate human rights and provide guidance in relation to the progressive realisation of particular rights. Relevant groups include refugees, asylum seekers, as well as the specialised convention in relation to disabled people. General Comment 14 (CESCR 2000) provides extensive guidance on the right to the highest attainable standard of health and on how this is to be interpreted, including defining the core obligations or minimum level in terms of essential primary health care, as discussed in Chapter 2. There has also been work on appropriate information/indicators for monitoring health equity, Bambas's (2005) paper on a human rights approach to health and information, and work on indicators for monitoring achievement of the right to health (Backman *et al.* 2008).

Reproductive health is another area where human rights have proved particularly influential, first of all in supporting the development of an appropriate understanding of reproductive health. The definition first formulated by WHO in 1987–8 was adopted, expanded and developed through two important conferences: the International Conference on Population and Development (ICPD) held in Cairo in 1994 and International Conference on Women held in Beijing in 1995:

> Reproductive health is a state of complete physical, mental and social well-being and not merely the absence of disease or infirmity, in all matters relating to the reproductive system and to its functions and processes. Reproductive health therefore implies that people are able to have a satisfying and safe sex life and that they have the capability to reproduce and the freedom to decide if, when and how often to do so. Implicit in this last condition are the right of men and women to be informed and to have access to safe, effective, affordable and acceptable methods of family planning of their choice, as well as other methods of their choice for regulation of fertility which are not against the law, and the right of access to appropriate health-care services that will enable women to go safely through pregnancy and childbirth and provide couples with the best chance of having a healthy infant.
>
> (UNFPA 1994: para 7.2)

In line with the above definition of reproductive health, reproductive health care is defined as the constellation of methods, techniques and services that contribute to reproductive health and wellbeing by preventing and solving reproductive health problems. It also includes sexual health, the purpose of which is the enhancement of life and personal relations, and not merely counselling and care related to reproduction and sexually transmitted diseases. Many different variants of the definition exist, reflecting the fact that this is remains a highly contested area. See for example Maticka-Tyndale and Smylie (2008) for a discussion of some of the debates with respect to sexual rights. Some leave out mention of 'which are not against the law'; some leave out mention of 'safe and satisfying sex life'. Note also that the definition implies that all sexes have reproductive rights. Despite the progress made in the years to 1995, sexual and reproductive health remains a contested area that suffers from lack of recognition and underfunding (Glasier and Gülmezoglu 2006), with many challenges, but also potential solutions (Davies 2010). The latest report from the current special rapporteur on the right to health (Grover 2011) illustrates the many negative effects that laws and other legal restrictions have on sexual and reproductive health globally, and call for measures to decriminalise abortion, the supply and use of all forms of contraception, and provision of information relating to sexual and reproductive health, as well as a range of other recommendations.

Human rights may benefit work in the area of public health by providing consistent guidance to states as human rights cross-cut all United Nations activities

A number of particular topics and groups provide evidence of where this particular benefit of human rights has been realised. It is clearly apparent in the case of HIV/AIDS. Production of specific guidance on human rights and involuntary detention for extensively drug-resistant tuberculosis control (WHO 2007b) has also been of importance. Another related area is that of access to pharmaceuticals and to essential medicines in particular (Lazzarini 2003; Lage 2011). Finally, in terms of particular population groups, work on access to services for disadvantaged groups and the health of women, refugees, asylum seekers and children has benefited from human rights approaches, as discussed throughout earlier chapters. Much still remains to be done however. The High Commissioner for Human Rights recognises this explicitly in discussion of the work that needs to continue on the programme of mainstreaming human rights in all UN activities (OHCHR 2011a) that was initiated by Kofi Annan during his time as Secretary-General in his programme for reform delivered to the General Assembly in July 1997 (UN Doc. A/51/950).

Human rights may benefit work in the area of public health by providing increased scope of analysis and range of partners in countries

The final element in WHO's list of value added can be evidenced in the work of a number of different campaigns and networks. In terms of international scope, two examples are provided by the People's Health Movement (PHM) and their work around the right to health, and second by international work around HIV/AIDS.

PHM was founded, after a year's preparatory work by an international network of activist organisations and NGOs, during the first People's Health Assembly, held in 2000 in Bangladesh (Baum 2001; Turiano and Smith 2008). During this Assembly, the People's Charter for Health, a previously drafted document, was finalised by the Assembly. The Charter has since become the most widely endorsed consensus document on health since the Alma Ata Declaration (Turiano and Smith 2008). The PHM is an international network of individuals and organisations, grouping together by country into so-called PHM circles. Initial work by the PHM concentrated on putting primary health care back on the agenda. The Women's Access to Health Campaign was launched in 2003 by Women's Global Network for Reproductive Rights (WGNRR) in collaboration with PHM to raise awareness and strengthen efforts to promote women's health with a primary health care approach. The PHM's Right to Health and Health Care Campaign was launched in 2005, and involves coordinated national- and international-level action. The first phase in this campaign involves the production of rights-based evaluations of national health policies in countries with PHM circles, using the assessment tool developed by PHM members (PHM 2006). These assessments will then form the basis for advocacy at country, regional and global levels.

Turiano and Smith (2008) describe how the right to health campaign developed out of the experience of one of the PHM circles, that of India, who started running a national Right to Health Care Campaign in 2003 and pioneered the strategic use of a right to health and health care framework to fight deterioration of the Indian public health system. The documentation produced was presented to the Indian National Human Rights Commission who then worked with them to produce a National Action Plan to Operationalise the Right to Health. Another example at country level is given by Khoo (2012), who examines the successes of the Consumers' Association of Penang in Malaysia, in its work on local and global health rights. Their alternative consumer approach distinctively integrates health with development, social justice and environmental issues. While not always explicitly employing rights language, the organisation has served as a powerful node in networked consumer campaigns to contest and shape global health governance.

Finally, a variety of international work in relation to HIV/AIDS has been discussed throughout earlier chapters in this book. A quote from the 2006 World Conference on AIDS taken from Amnesty International's public statement issued on 18 August 2006, illustrates how central human rights has become in work on HIV/AIDS:

> As the XVI International AIDS Conference in Toronto comes to an end, Amnesty International issues an urgent call to governments and to the international community to place human rights at the centre of responses to HIV/AIDS. Twenty-five years into the epidemic the need for human rights based approaches to HIV/AIDS cannot go unheeded any longer. Debates at the conference – whose theme was 'Time to deliver' – highlighted the extent

to which human rights approaches are indivisible from successful public health policy. ... Only by respecting human rights can we ensure success in the equitable scaling–up to universal access to treatment, care and prevention.

The value of rights-based approaches

Looking back over the different chapters in this book, a wealth of examples can be seen of positive effects of the use of rights-based approaches at international, regional, national and local levels in terms of policy formulation and the design, implementation and evaluation of specific programmes and activities. The examples considered cover the whole range of countries at different stages of development, and in particular have focused attention on the most disadvantaged or marginalised groups. One of the reasons underlying such success is identified by Jonsson (2003) who explicitly compares needs-based approaches to human rights-based approaches in the context of development planning, noting that:

> Although human rights are need-based claims, a human rights approach to programming differs sharply from the basic needs approach. Most importantly, the basic needs approach does not imply the existence of a duty-bearer. When demands for meeting needs have no 'object,' nobody has a clear-cut duty to meet needs, and rights are vulnerable to ongoing violation.
>
> (Jonsson 2003: 20)

It is important to acknowledge however that RBAs are not a 'magic wand' to be waved to solve all problems. As Crammond has illustrated in Chapter 11, RBAs do not provide solutions in terms of difficult resources allocation decisions between competing health problems and target groups, although they may well help define appropriate processes by which such decisions can be reached. A further critical look at dangers and difficulties of RBAs is provided by Davis (2009) in his analysis of rights-based approaches to development.

Necessary complexity or needless bureaucracy?

This book has also examined the various human rights systems that exist, global, regional and national, a complex interacting system of systems with multiple points of interaction and leverage. At first sight, this can be confusing and certainly not straightforward to navigate as an individual or group with a human rights concern. However, this complexity allows for multiple points of influence and leverage that do, in particular circumstances, assist in addressing human rights issues. Japan, which does not connect directly into any regional human rights system, and without a national human rights institution, nonetheless has been influenced within the international system, as was discussed in Chapter 4. In terms of regional and global systems, it has been suggested that in some cases countries, particularly newly emerged democracies, have agreed to participate in such systems as a way to consolidate, or 'lock in', recent domestic democratic reforms. International human rights bodies can operate in a range of ways to prevent reversion into authoritarian practices, and are therefore a useful tool for newly democratic governments who face internal challenges (both actual and anticipated) to their democratic gains (Munro 2009). This theory was first suggested by Moravcsik (2000), and his examination of the European Convention of Human Rights showed supportive evidence. However Simmons (2002) in her study of six UN human rights treaties (CAT, CEDAW, CRC, ICCPR, ICESCR and ICERD) finds most evidence of socialisation through persuasion from actors external to the country which she calls 'external socialisation', rather than pressure by powerful state actors or democratic lock-in. Similarly Munro in his study of the creation of the AICHR (Munro 2009) concludes that regional groupings may nowadays find it 'appropriate' or 'necessary' to construct human rights regimes to remain active participants in the international community. They may fear a 'pariah status' and even sanctions if they do not participate in the established international discourse on human rights.

The UN: a conflicted organisation

Charged with promoting and protecting human rights, including the right to health, the UN is faced with difficulty in doing this in the face of the current neoliberal global finance and trade mechanisms, adhered to by its own agencies. The actions of the World Bank, the International Monetary Fund and the World Trade Organization directly sustain many human rights violations, see Macdonald (2008) and Stiglitz (2006). A major challenge for the organisation is to try to address the tensions this causes, hopefully with the result of reaffirming human rights as the central principle for the operation of all the UN agencies. While documenting considerable criticism of the UN, Macdonald (2008) rejects the conclusion that the UN should be abandoned; instead he argues for its reform, in both organisational and philosophical terms, placing human rights at the centre of all its operations; Fox and Meier (2009) argue that focusing on the collective human right to development would prove a more powerful legal framework to create a just and equitable international economic order for the improvement of health in developing countries, and that this would support improvements in the whole array of social determinants of health.

In terms of the right to health in particular, Macdonald (2007) argues that under present global economic models, global equity in health is impossible, and achieving the right to health requires the adoption of an alternative economic paradigm; he identifies promising avenues in the use of international health impact assessments and regional fair trade zones. In this context ongoing debates about global health governance are particularly important (Ng and Ruger 2011). Ongoing concern is being expressed about the impact of trade agreements on health. For example, Gleeson (2011) discusses the Trans Pacific Partnership Agreement currently under negotiation, which US corporations are trying to use to achieve advantageous terms that may protect their profits, but at the cost of reducing access to essential medicines. The most recent annual report of the High Commissioner for Human Rights (OHCHR 2011a) discusses the need to strengthen the UN human rights system, especially in the light of the increases in the size of the system (doubling in the time from 2004 to 2010), and is in the midst of a consultation process regarding how this is to be achieved.

Looking to the future: opportunities and challenges

Many challenges still remain, first and foremost perhaps is that of ensuring that RBAs are used to their full effect for public health purposes, especially in the demanding socio-political context consequent on the 'Arab Spring', and the health threats posed by climate change. Even in HIV/AIDS, the field in which rights-based approaches started to be developed and honed, considerable work needs still to be done to tackle rights violations for specific population groups, see for example Center for Reproductive Rights and Vivo Positivo (2010), based on research conducted in 2009–10, who document the systemic discrimination and abuse that HIV-positive women experience in Chilean health facilities, and Kendall (2009) on the experience of HIV-positive Mexican women. OHCHR (2011a) identifies that around fifty countries impose some form of restriction on entry, stay or residence based on people's HIV status alone. The latest report by the UN Secretary-General on HIV/AIDS (UN Secretary-General 2011) acknowledges the stigma, discrimination and gender inequality that continue to undermine efforts to achieve universal access to HIV prevention, treatment, care and support, and calls for a continued focus on human rights as a part of the solution. Calls for the use of rights-based approaches are becoming more widespread, for tackling issues as diverse as cervical cancer in Africa (Durojaye *et al.* 2011) and access to services for homeless families in England (Stuttaford *et al.* 2009).

Felner (2009) argues that a further challenge remains in terms of monitoring progressive realisation of economic, social and cultural rights. Progressive realisation in the terms of the ICESCR is expressed, qualified by 'to the maximum of the state's available resources', and this brings into play questions of resource prioritisation. Felner argues that monitoring methods that focus on this area could provide powerful tools for social change, and sets out a three-step framework within which such monitoring could be located. It remains to be seen whether such an approach, and the more sophisticated methods he overviews briefly, including the use of econometric tools and economic models, are taken up by human rights activists and/or NHRIs.

Trends in increasing development of NHRIs have been mentioned as well as their increased integration into the UN system; the full implications of this remain to be explored in the future. There is also an increased emphasis on citizen education on human rights and on the further potential of human rights defenders. To support this there are growing sections of the OHCHR website on human rights education. Accompanying this is the growing production of guides and resource books for use by concerned individuals, human rights defenders or activists. For example, at global level, AHRC (2011) is a guide to using the Optional Protocol to CEDAW and other international complaint mechanisms; OHCHR (2008) is a handbook for civil society on working with the United Nations Human Rights Programme; Asher (2004) is a resource manual for NGOs on the right to health; and Asher *et al.* (2007) is a tool kit for health professionals on the right to health and their day-today work. There are also regional and national guides, for example, Kagoiya (2009) on women's rights in Africa, MacNeil (2011) on rights work with local government in South Africa and Tiwana *et al.* (2006) on Human Rights Commissions in India. Alongside this, an increasing discussion of human rights fieldwork as a profession can be identified (see e.g. O'Flaherty and Ulrich 2010).

The links between human rights and the social determinants of health are becoming increasingly recognised; Blas *et al.* (2011) examine social determinants approaches to public health and provide many examples of where programmes and initiatives have justified their activities in terms of achievements of particular rights, and in some cases (Hargreaves *et al.* 2011) have used explicitly rights-based approaches. A recent publication by ILO (2011: 6) takes up the question of the 'pivotal role of freedom of association in fostering and maintaining sustainable development', and illustrating this through examples taken from areas such as inclusive economic growth and poverty reduction, positive business environments, crisis response, and finally democracy and governance. Rasanathan *et al.* (2010) provide thoughtful discussions of some of the challenges and opportunities in taking this work further in the future.

Rights-based approaches have a potentially highly significant role to play in global health governance. As Ng and Ruger (2011) note, the state of global health governance evidenced in the literature is one beset by the continuance of problems such as insufficient coordination, dominance of narrow national and or organisational self-interest, insufficient participation and resource shortage. Ooms (2011) analyses the global response to HIV/AIDS and argues that there is scope for developing a global social contract for health with its basis in the right to health. The WHO European Regional Office for Europe sees human rights as providing the 'value frame' within which its new regional health policy, Health 2020, will sit (EURO 2011). Finally, a coalition of civil society organisations and academics has initiated a programme of work aimed at securing a global health agreement and supporting social mobilisation around the right to health (Gostin *et al.* 2011).

So, at the end of this book, it should be clear that rights-based approaches do not represent a magic wand to ensure universal achievement of human rights and the removal of health inequity under all circumstances. However, very many different examples of where rights-based approaches have been useful have been identified, as well as other examples where success has been more qualified. As the work of CARE International discussed at some length in Chapter 5 explicitly demonstrated, there may well be situations where it is not considered appropriate to use the language of rights.

Although human rights-based approaches do not provide the response to every challenge, they may represent one of the most useful frameworks we have in meeting the challenge of health inequities globally, nationally and at local levels. The challenge for the future is to continue to develop these, and to disseminate them widely, both amongst health and social care/welfare professionals and amongst the general population. It remains to be seen exactly how far the potential provided by rights-based approaches can assist public health practitioners in working for health and social justice.

Notes on sources

In discussing the basic history and structures of human rights systems, use has been made of websites and a few key references. Rather than compromise the readability of the text by attempting to reference each point explicitly, basic notes on these sources are provided here.

General sources used throughout to check details of basic documentation and dates

- *A Thematic Guide to Documents on Health and Human Rights* (Alfredsson and Tomasevski 1998)
- *Human Rights: Treaties, Statutes and Cases* (Flynn et al. 2011)
- *The Wilson Chronology of Human Rights* (Levinson 2003)
- *Health and Human Rights: Basic International Documents* (Marks 2005)
- *Human Rights: A Compilation of International Instruments* (UN Centre for Human Rights 1994–7)

Chapter 2

- www.ohchr.org
- *The United Nations and Human Rights: A Guide for a New Era* (Mertus 2009)
- *The United Nations Human Rights System* (OHCHR n.d.)
- *Human Rights: A Compilation of International Instruments* (UN Centre for Human Rights 1994–7)

NGOs in the global system

Websites as listed in Table 2.6. Recent annual reports: HRW (2011); MSF (2010); Amnesty International (2011).

Chapter 3

Africa

- http://www.achpr.org – website of African Commission on Human and Peoples' Rights

- http://www.african-court.org – website of African Court on Human and Peoples' Rights
- http://www.au.int – website of the African Union
- *The African Human Rights System* (Kufuor 2010)

Americas

- http://www.cidh.oas.org – website of the Inter-American Commission on Human Rights
- http://www.oas.org/en/default.asp – website of the Organization of American States
- http://www.corteidh.or.cr – website of the Inter-American Court of Human Rights

Asia-Pacific

- http://www.aseansec.org/ – website of ASEAN
- http://www.forum-asia.org/ – website of Forum-Asia

Europe

- http://www.echr.coe.int/ECHR – website of the European Court of Human Rights
- http://echr.coe.int/echr/en/hudoc – portal for public information sources at the ECHR
- http://fra.europa.eu/fraWebsite/home/home_en.htm – website of the European Union Agency for Fundamental Rights (FRA)
- http://www.eucharter.org – website covering the history and development of the EU Charter of Fundamental Rights
- http://ec.europa.eu – website of the European Commission
- http://ec.europa.eu/justice/fundamental-rights – website for rights within the Department of Justice at the European Commission

Middle East and Organisation of Islamic Cooperation

- www.arableagueonline.org – website of the League of Arab States
- http://www.cihrs.org – website of the Cairo Institute for Human Rights Studies, independent regional NGO founded in 1993
- http://www.oic-oci.org – website of OIC

Chapter 4

Sweden

- http://www.humanrights.gov.se – website of Swedish government on human rights

- http://www.do.se/en – website of equality ombudsman, 'Diskrimineringsombudsmannen' (DO)

Ghana

The Parliament of Ghana is in the process of launching a new website. The old website that was used has not been maintained. The CHRAJ website was part of the website.

Australia

- http://www.humanrights.gov.au – website of the Australian Human Rights Commission
- http://www.humanrightscommission.vic.gov.au – website of the Victorian Equal Opportunity and Human Rights Commission
- *The Politics of Human Rights in Australia* (Chappell et al. 2009)

India

- http://www.nhrc.nic.in/ – website of the National Human Rights Commission, New Delhi

Japan

- http://www.moj.go.jp/ENGLISH/HB/hb.html – website of the Japanese Ministry of Justice Human Rights Bureau
- http://www.hurights.or.jp/english – website of Human Rights Osaka, the Asia-Pacific Human Rights Information Center opened in 1994, supported by Osaka prefecture, Osaka city, several non-governmental organisations and various other organisations and individuals

National Human Rights Institutions

- http://nhri.ohchr.org/

Chapter 5

CARE International case study – material from CARE International UK's website.

Chapter 12

History and development of the PHM from material on their website.

References

ABS (2009) *Experimental Life Tables for Aboriginal and Torres Strait Islander Australians, 2005–2007, 3302.0.55.003*, Canberra: Australian Bureau of Statistics.
ACER (2010) *MindMatters Evaluation Report Submitted to Principals Australia*, Camberwell, Vic.: ACER, Australian Council for Educational Research.
ACHPR (2001) *Communication 155/96: The Social and Economic Rights Action Center and the Center for Economic and Social Rights/Nigeria*, Banjul: ACHPR.
ACHPR (2003) *Communication 241/01: Purohit and Moore/The Gambia*. Banjul: ACHPR.
ACHPR (2008) *Consideration of Reports submitted by States Parties under Article 62 of the African Charter of Human and Peoples' Rights: Concluding Observations and Recommendations on the Third Periodic Report of the Federal Republic of Nigeria*, 44th ordinary session, 10–24 Nov., Abuja: Nigeria.
African Court on Human and Peoples' Rights (2011) *In the matter of the African Commission on Human and Peoples' Rights vs the Great Libyan Peoples' Arab Jamahiraya, Application number 004/2011 Order for Provisional Measures*, Arusha: African Court on Human and Peoples' Rights.
Afridi, F. (2005) 'Mid day meals: a comparison of the financial and institutional organization of the program in two states', *Economic and Political Weekly*, 40(15): 1529–34.
AFRO (2009) *WHO Country Cooperation Strategy 2008–2013 Gambia*, Brazzaville: WHO Regional Office for Africa.
Aggleton, P. (1997) *Success in HIV Prevention: Some Strategies and Approaches*, Horsham, West Sussex: AVERT.
Agha, S. (2002) 'An evaluation of the effectiveness of a peer sexual health intervention among secondary school students in Zambia', *AIDS Education and Prevention*, 14: 269–81.
AHRC (2009) *Human Rights Explained: Fact Sheet 2: Human Rights Origins*. Canberra: Australian Human Rights Commission.
AHRC (2010a) *Australian Human Rights Commission Annual Report 2009–2010*, Sydney: Australian Human Rights Commission.
AHRC (2010b) *In our own Words – African Australians: A Review of Human Rights and Social Inclusion Issues*, Sydney: Australian Human Rights Commission.
AHRC (2010c) *Gender Equality Blueprint 2010*, Sydney: Australian Human Rights Commission.
AHRC (2011) *Mechanisms for Advancing Women's Human Rights: A Guide to Using the Optional Protocol to CEDAW and Other International Complaint Mechanisms*, Sydney: AHRC.
AIDA and CHETRE (2010) *Health Impact Assessment of the Northern Territory Emergency Response*, Canberra: Australian Indigenous Doctors' Association.

Aim for Human Rights (2008) *Health Rights of Women Assessment Instrument*, Utrecht: Aim for Human Rights.

Ainley, J., Withers, G., Underwood, C., and Frigo, T. (2006) *National Survey of Health and Well-Being Promotion Policies and Practice in Secondary Schools*, Melbourne: Australian Council for Educational Research.

Alfredsson, G., and Tomasevski, K., eds (1998) *A Thematic Guide to Documents on Health and Human Rights: Global and Regional Standards Adopted by Intergovernmental Organizations, International Non-Governmental Organizations, and Professional Associations*, The Hague and London: M. Nijhoff.

Alsop, R., ed. (2004) *Power, Rights, and Poverty: Concepts and Connections,* a working meeting sponsored by DFID and the World Bank, Washington, DC, and London: World Bank/DFID.

Amnesty International (2011) *Amnesty International Report 2010: The State of the World's Human Rights*, London: Amnesty International.

Amunwa, B. (2011) *Counting the Cost: Corporations and Human Rights Abuses in the Niger Delta*, London: Platform.

Anderson, T. (2009) 'HIV/AIDS in Cuba: a rights-based analysis', *Health and Human Rights in Practice*, 11(1): 93–104.

Annette, J., and Mayo, M., eds (2010) *Taking Part? Active Learning for Active Citizenship, and Beyond,* London: NIACE.

Armstrong, K. (2002) 'Spirituality, health, stolen generation(s) and reconciliation with our indigenous peoples: childhood – the missing dimension', *Aboriginal and Islander Health Worker Journal*, 26(5): 26–9.

ASEAN (2009) *ASEAN Intergovernmental Commission on Human Rights: Terms of Reference*, Jakarta: ASEAN.

Asher, J. (2004) *The Right to Health: A Resource Manual for NGOs*, London: Commonwealth Medical Trust.

Asher, J., Hamm, D., and Sheather, J. (2007) *The Right to Health: A Toolkit for Health Professionals*, London: British Medical Association.

Asibuo, S. K. (2001) *The Role of the Commission on Human Rights and Administrative Justice (CHRAJ) in Promoting Public Service Accountability under Ghana's Fourth Republic*, Tangier: African Training and Research Centre in Administration for Development.

Askell-Williams, H., Lawson, M., Murray-Harvey, R., and Slee, P. (2005) *An Investigation of the Implementation of a MindMatters Teaching Module in Secondary School Classrooms*, Adelaide: School of Education, Flinders University.

Backman, G., Hunt, P., Khosla, R., Jaramillo-Strouss, C., Fikre, B. M., Rumble, C., Pevalin, D., Páez, D. A., Pineda, M. A., Frisancho, A., Tarco, D., Motlagh, M., Farcasanu, D., and Vladescu, C. (2008) 'Health systems and the right to health: an assessment of 194 countries', *The Lancet*, 372(9655): 2047–85.

Bajaj, M. (2012) 'From "time pass" to transformative force: school-based human rights education in Tamil Nadu, India', *International Journal of Educational Development,* 32(1): 72–80.

Bajpai, N., Sachs, J. D., and Dholakia, R. H. (2010) *Improving Access and Efficiency in Public Health Services: Mid-Term Evaluation of India's National Rural Health Mission*, New Delhi: Sage.

Bakker, S., Van Den Berg, M., Düzenli, D., and Radstaake, M. (2009) 'Human rights impact assessment in practice: the case of the Health Rights of Women Assessment Instrument (HeRWAI)', *Journal of Human Rights Practice*, 1(3): 436–58.

Bambas, L. (2005) 'Integrating equity into health information systems: a human rights approach to health and information', *PLoS Medicine*, 2: 299–301.

Bankston, C. L., III (2010) 'Social justice: cultural origins of a theory and a perspective', *Independent Review*, 15(2): 165–78.

Barron, P., and Roma-Reardon, J., eds (2008) *South African Health Review 2008*, Health Systems Trust: www.hst.org.za/publications/8419 (accessed April 2009).

Barsh, R. L. (1996) 'Indigenous peoples and the UN Commission on Human Rights: a case of the immovable object and the irresistible force', *Human Rights Quarterly*, 18: 782–813.

Batra, A., and Buchkremer, G. (2004) *Tabakentwöhnung: Ein Leitfaden für Therapeuten*, Stuttgart: Kohlhammer.

Baum, F. (1998) *The New Public Health*, Oxford: Oxford University Press.

Baum, F. (2001) 'Health, equity, justice and globalisation: some lessons from the People's Health Assembly', *Journal of Epidemiology and Community Health*, 55: 613–16.

Bauman, A. E., Fardy, H. J., and Harris, P. G. (2003) 'Getting it right: why bother with patient-centred care?', *Medical Journal of Australia*, 179(5): 253–6.

Bayley, O. (2003) 'Improvement of sexual and reproductive health requires focusing on adolescents', *The Lancet*, 362: 830–1.

Bearinger, L. H., Sieving, R. E., Ferguson, J., and Sharma, V. (2007) 'Global perspectives on the sexual and reproductive health of adolescents: patterns, prevention and potential', *The Lancet*, 369: 1220–31.

Beauchamp, D. E. (1976) 'Public health as social justice', *Inquiry*, 13(1): 3–14.

Bedford, J., Marsh, H., and Wright, D. (2006) *The National Framework for Active Learning for Active Citizenship*, London: Togetherwecan.

Beer, C., and Mitchell, N. J. (2006) 'Comparing nations and states: human rights and democracy in India', *Comparative Political Studies,* 39(8): 996–1018.

Berman, G. (2008) *Undertaking a Human Rights-Based Approach: A Guide for Basic Programming – Documenting Lessons Learned for Human Rights-Based Programming. An Asia-Pacific Perspective: Implications for Policy, Planning and Programming*, Bangkok: UNESCO.

Bernardi, G. (2001) 'From conflict to convergence: the evolution of Tasmanian anti-discrimination law', *Australian Journal of Human Rights,* 6: www.austlii.edu.au/au/journals/AJHR/2001/6.html.

Bhagavan, M. (2010) 'A new hope: India, the United Nations and the making of the universal declaration of human rights', *Modern Asian Studies,* 44(2): 311–47.

Bickenbach, J. E. (2009) 'Disability, culture and the UN convention', *Disability and Rehabilitation*, 31(14): 1111–24.

Birgden, A., and Cucolo, H. (2011) 'The treatment of sex offenders: evidence, ethics and human rights', *Sexual Abuse: Journal of Research and Treatment*, 23(3): 295–313.

Bisaillon, L. M. (2010) 'Human rights consequences of mandatory HIV screening policy of newcomers to Canada', *Health and Human Rights,* 12(2): 119–34.

Black Sash (2011) *Making Human Rights Real: Report on Nine Provincial Community Consultations on Health Reform*, Cape Town: Atlantic Philanthropies.

Blas, E., Sommerfeld, J., and Kurup, A. S., eds (2011) *Social Determinants Approaches to Public Health: From Concept to Practice*, Geneva: WHO.

Bolis, M. (2002) *The Impact of the Caracas Declaration on the Modernization of Mental Health Legislation in Latin America and the English-speaking Caribbean*, Washington D.C.: PAHO.

Bond, L., Glover, S., Godfrey, C., Butler, H., and Patton, G. C. (2001) 'Building capacity for system-level change in schools: lessons from the Gatehouse Project', *Health Education and Behaviour*, 28(3): 368–83.

Braveman, P., and Gruskin, S. (2003a) 'Poverty, equity, human rights and health', *Bulletin of the World Health Organization*, 81: 539–45.

Braveman, P., and Gruskin, S. (2003b) 'Defining equity in health', *Journal of Epidemiology and Community Health*, 57: 254–8.

Bringing Them Home (1997) *Bringing Them Home: Report of the National Inquiry into the Separation of Aboriginal and Torres Strait Islander Children from their Families*, Sydney: Commonwealth of Australia.

Brinton Lykes, M. (2001) 'Human rights violations as structural violence', in D. J. Christie, R. V. Wagner and D. A. Winter (eds), *Peace, Conflict, and Violence: Peace Psychology for the 21st Century*, Englewood Cliffs, NJ: Prentice-Hall.

Broderstad, E. G. (2010) 'Indigenous rights and citizenship rights: contradictory or coherent?', presentation at the 11th annual Forum for Development Cooperation with Indigenous Peoples, 24–6 Oct., Centre for Sámi Studies, University of Tromsø, Norway. Full conference report available in Munin at http://hdl.handle.net/10037/2941.

Brough, M., Gorman, D., Ramirez, E., and Westoby, P. (2003) 'Young refugees talk about well-being: a qualitative analysis of refugee youth mental health from three states', *Australian Journal of Social Issues*, 38(2): 193–208.

Brugha, R., and Varvasovsky, Z. (2000) 'Stakeholder analysis: a review', *Health Policy and Planning*, 15: 239–46.

Brundtland, G. H. (2005) 'The UDHR: fifty years of synergy between health and human rights', in S. Gruskin, M. Grodin, S. Marks and G. Annas (eds), *Perspectives on Health and Human Rights*, New York: Routledge.

Brühler, A., and Kröger, C. (2006) *Expertise zur Prävention des Substanzmissbrauchs, Forschung und Praxis der Gesundheitsförderung*, vol. 29, Cologne: Bundeszentrale für gesundheitliche Aufklärung.

Butler, D. (2004) 'Health experts find obesity measures too lightweight', *Nature*, 428: 244.

Cabal, L., Roa, M., and Sepúlveda-Oliva, L. (2003) 'What role can international litigation play in the promotion and advancement of reproductive rights in Latin America?' *Health and Human Rights*, 7(1): 51–88.

Calma, T. (2008) 'Ten years on: life chances and human rights of indigenous children', *Reform*, 92: 13–17.

Campbell, C., Foulis, C. A., Maimane, S., and Sibiya, Z. (2005) 'The impact of social environments on the effectiveness of youth HIV prevention: a South African case study', *AIDS Care*, 17: 471–8.

Canning, U., Millward, L., Raj, T., and Warm, D. (2004) *Drug Use Prevention among Young People: A Review of Reviews*, London: Health Development Agency.

Carver, R. (2010) 'A new answer to an old question: national human rights institutions and the domestication of international law', *Human Rights Law Review*, 10(1): 1–32.

Carver, R. (2011) 'One NHRI or Many? How Many Institutions does it Take to Protect Human Rights? Lessons from the European Experience', *Journal of Human Rights Practice*, 3(1): 1–24.

Castellano, M. B., Archibald, L., and DeGagné, M. (2008) *From Truth to Reconciliation: Transforming the Legacy of Residential Schools*, Ottawa: Aboriginal Healing Foundation.

Center for Reproductive Rights and Vivo Positivo (2010) *Dignity Denied: Violations of the Rights of HIV-Positive Women in Chilean Health Facilities,* New York: Center for Reproductive Rights.

Centre for Human Rights (1994) *Human Rights and Social Work: A Manual for Schools of Social Work and the Social Work Profession*, Professional Training Series, 1, Geneva: United Nations.

CESCR (1990) *General Comment No. 3: The Nature of State Parties' Obligations*, Geneva: United Nations.
CESCR (2000) *General Comment No. 14: The Right to the Highest Attainable Standard of Health*, Geneva: United Nations.
CESCR (2001) 'Human rights and intellectual property', in Committee on Economic, Social and Cultural Rights, *Report on the 25th, 26th and 27th Sessions*, UN Doc. E/2002/22–E/C.I2/2001/1/I7, Annex XIII, Geneva: UN.
Chapman, A. R. (2010) 'The social determinants of health, health equity, and human rights', *Health and Human Rights*, 12(2): 17–30.
Chapman, J. (1990) 'Violence Against Women as a Violation of Human Rights', *Social Justice*, 17(2).
Chapman, J., and Mancini, A., eds (2006) *Critical Webs of Power and Change: A Resource Pack for Planning, Assessment and Learning in People-Centred Advocacy*, Johannesburg: ActionAid.
Chapman, S. (1993) 'Unravelling gossamer with boxing gloves: problems in explaining the decline in smoking', *British Medical Journal*, 307: 429–32.
Chappell, L., Chesterman, J., and Hill, L. (2009) *The Politics of Human Rights in Australia*, Port Melbourne: Cambridge University Press.
Chettiparamb, A. (2009) 'Policy build-up in implementation: the case of school meals provision in Kodungallur, Kerala, India', *European Journal of Development Research*. 21: 419–34.
Chettiparambil-Rajan, A. (2007) *A Desk Review of the Mid-Day Meals Programme,* Rome: World Food Programme: http://home.wfp.org/stellent/groups/public/documents/newsroom/wfp207424.pdf (accessed May 2010).
Chopra, M., and Ford, N. (2005) 'Scaling up health promotion interventions in the era of HIV/AIDS: challenges for a rights based approach', *Health Promotion International*, 20(4): 383–90.
CHRAJ (2008) *Submission of UPR report to the UN HRC*, Accra: CHRAJ.
CIHRS (2008) *Human Rights in the Arab Region: Annual Report 2008*, Cairo: Cairo Institute for Human Rights Studies.
CIHRS (2010) *Roots of Unrest: Human Rights in the Arab Region. Annual Report 2010*, Cairo: Cairo Institute for Human Rights Studies.
Claude, R. P., and Issel, B. W. (1998) 'Health, medicine and science in the drafting of the Universal Declaration of Human Rights', *Health and Human Rights*, 3(2): 126–42.
Coker, R. (2001) 'Just coercion? Detention of nonadherent tuberculosis patients', *Annals of the New York Academy of Sciences*, 953: 216–23.
Cook, R., Dickens, B., and Fathalla, M. (2003) *Reproductive Health and Human Rights: Integrating Medicine, Ethics and Law*, Oxford: Clarendon Press.
Commission on Human Rights (2001) *Access to Medication in the Context of Pandemics such as HIV/AIDS, Resolution 2001/53*, Geneva: OHCHR.
Coulter, A., and Collins, A. (2011) *Making Shared Decision-Making a Reality: No Decision About Me, Without Me*, London: King's Fund.
Couzos, S., and Thiele, D. D. (2007) 'The ICESCR and the right to health: is Australia meeting its obligations to Aboriginal peoples?' *Medical Journal of Australia*, 186(10): 522–4.
CRC (2000) *Concluding Observations of the Committee on the Rights of the Child: South Africa*, United Nations: www.unhchr.ch/tbs/doc.nsf/%20 (Symbol)/CRC.C.15.Add.122.En?Opendocument (retrieved April 2009).
CSDH (2008) *Closing the Gap in a Generation: Health Equity through Action on the Social Determinants of Health*, Geneva: World Health Organization.

Cullet, P. (2003) 'Patents and medicines: the relationship between TRIPS and the human right to health', *International Affairs*, 79(1): 139–60.
Curtice, M. J., and Exworthy, T. (2010) 'FREDA: A human rights-based approach to healthcare', *Psychiatrist*, 34(4): 150–6.
Daniels, N. (2008) *Just Health: Meeting Health Needs Fairly*, New York: Cambridge University Press.
Davies, S. E. (2010) 'Reproductive health as a human right: a matter of access or provision?', *Journal of Human Rights*, 9(4): 387–408.
Davis, T. W. D. (2009) 'The politics of human rights and development: the challenge for official donors', *Australian Journal of Political Science*, 44(1): 173–92.
De Cock, K. M., Mbori-Ngacha, D., and Marum, E. (2002) 'Shadow on the continent: public health and HIV/AIDS in Africa in the 21st century', *The Lancet*, 360: 67–72.
De Negri Filho, A. (2008) 'A human rights approach to quality of life and health: applications to public health programming', *Health and Human Rights*, 10(1): 93–101.
de Vos, P., de Ceukelaire, W., Malaise, G., Perez, D., Lefevre, P., and van der Stuyft, P. (2009) 'Health through people's empowerment: a rights-based approach to participation', *Health and Human Rights*, 11(1): 23–35.
Department of Education and Early Childhood Development (2007) *At School 5–18*: www.education.vic.gov.au/aboutschool/default.htm (retrieved June 2009).
Department of Health (2007) *Human Rights in Healthcare: A Framework for Local Action*, London: Department of Health.
Department of Health and Ageing (2000) 'Minister releases youth mental health report': www.health.gov.au/internet/main/publishing.nsf/Content/health-mediarel-yr2000-mw-mw20124.htm (retrieved May 2009).
Department of Health and Ageing (2007) *National Mental Health Report 2007: Summary of Twelve Years of Reform in Australia's Mental Health Services under the National Mental Health Strategy 1993–2005*, Canberra: Commonwealth of Australia.
Department of Human Services (2000) *Evidence-Based Health Promotion: Resources for Planning*, no. 2, *Adolescent Health*, Victoria: Department of Human Services.
Department of Justice (2006) *The Charter of Human Rights and Responsibilities*, Victoria: State Government.
DG1 (1998) *European Commission (DG1) Note on the WHO's Revised Drug Strategy, Doc No 1/D/3/BW D (98) (Oct 5 1998)*, Brussels: European Commission.
Diwan, R. (2009) *Effective Delivery and Total Food Safety Measures in Delhi*: www.educationforallinindia.com/best-practices-mid-day-meal-delhi-rashmi-diwan.pdf (accessed May 2010).
Donald, A., and Mottershaw, E. (2009) 'Evaluating the impact of human rights litigation on policy and practice: a case study of the UK', *Journal of Human Rights Practice*, 1(3): 339–61.
Donald, A. Mottershaw, E., Leach, P., and Watson, J. (2009) *Evaluating the Impact of Selected Cases under the Human Rights Act on Public Services Provision*, London: EHRC.
Donnelly, J. (1999) 'Human rights and Asian values: a defense of "western" universalism', in J. R. Bauer and D. A. Bell (eds), *The East Asian Challenge for Human Rights*, Cambridge: Cambridge University Press.
DRDA (2010) *Sampoorna Grameen Rozgar Yojana*: www.drdacachar.org/programs/sgry.asp (accessed May 2010).
Dresler, C., and Marks, S. (2006) 'The emerging human right to tobacco control', *Human Rights Quarterly*, 28: 559–651.
Drèze, J., and Goyal, A. (2003) 'Future of mid-day meals', *Economic and Political Weekly*, 38: 4673–83.

Drèze, J., and Kingdon, G. (2001) 'School participation in rural India', *Review of Development Economics*, 5: 1–24.

Durojaye, E., Sholola, O., and Ngwena, C. (2011) 'A human rights response to cervical cancer in Africa', *International Journal of Human Rights*, 15(3): 416–40.

Durrant, J. E. (2008) 'Physical punishment, culture, and rights: current issues for professionals', *Journal of Developmental and Behavioral Pediatrics*, 29(1): 55–66.

ECOSOC (1984) *U.N. Sub-Commission on Prevention of Discrimination and Protection of Minorities, Siracusa Principles on the Limitation and Derogation of Provisions in the International Covenant on Civil and Political Rights. UN Document E/CN.4/1984/4, Annex*, Geneva: UN.

Editors (1994) 'Gay Rights Victory at UN – I', *Human Rights Defender*, 1: www.ustlii.edu.au/au/journals/HRD/1994/1.html

Education for All in India (2010) *Mid-Day Meal Scheme*: http://education.nic.in/mdm/mdm1995.asp (accessed May 2010).

EHRC (2009a) *Human Rights Inquiry: Report of the Equality and Human Rights Commission*, London: EHRC.

EHRC (2009b) *The Impact of Human Rights Culture on Public Sector Organisations: Lessons from Practice*, London: EHRC.

EHRC (2009c) *The Role and Experience of Inspectorates, Regulators and Complaints-Handling Bodies in Promoting Human Rights Standards in Public Services: Final Report for the Equality and Human Rights Commission*, London: EHRC.

Eisenbruch, M., de Jong, J. V. M., and van de Put, W. (2004) 'Bringing order out of chaos: a culturally competent approach to managing the problems of refugees and victims of organised violence', *Journal of Traumatic Stress*, 17(2): 123–31.

EMRO (2006) *Human Rights in Support of the Right to Health: Report on an Intercountry Meeting on Health and Human Rights*, Cairo, Egypt, 12–14 July 2005, WHO-EM/ARD/025/E, Cairo: WHO Regional Office for the Eastern Mediterranean.

Encyclopaedia Britannica (2011) 'Permanent Arab Commission on Human Rights', in *Encyclopaedia Britannica*: www.britannica.com/EBchecked/topic/452208/Permanent-Arab-Commission-on-Human-Rights (accessed May 2011).

Equality Ombudsman (2010) *Gender Identity and Gender Expression*, Stockholm: Equality Ombudsman: www.do.se/Documents/Material/English/gender%20identity%20and%20gender%20expression%20tillganglig%20(2).pdf (accessed May 2011).

Equality Ombudsman (2011) *About the Equality Ombudsman*, Stockholm: Equality Ombudsman.

EU (2000) 'Charter of fundamental rights of the European Union', *Official Journal of the European Communities*, C364: 1–22.

EU Network (2006) *Commentary of the Charter of Fundamental Rights on the European Union*, Brussels: EU Network of Independent Experts on Human Rights.

EURO (2002) *European Strategy for Tobacco Control*, Copenhagen: WHO Regional Office for Europe.

EURO (2011) *Governance for Health in the 21st Century*, Copenhagen: WHO Regional Office for Europe, EUR/RC61/Inf.Doc./6.

European Court of Human Rights (2011) *Annual Report 2010 of the European Court of Human Rights, Council of Europe*, Strasbourg: Registry of the European Court of Human Rights.

Fagerström, K. (2002) 'The epidemiology of smoking: health consequences and benefits of cessation', *Drugs*, 62(suppl. 2): 1–9.

Farmer, P. (1999) 'Pathologies of power: rethinking health and human rights', *American Journal of Public Health*, 89(10): 1486–96.

Farmer, P. (2008) 'Challenging orthodoxies: the road ahead for health and human rights', *Health and Human Rights,* 10(1): 5–20.

Federal Ministry of Justice (2008) *Nigeria's Third Periodic Country Report 2005–2008 on the Implementation of the African Charter on Human and Peoples' Rights in Nigeria*, Abuja: Federal Ministry of Justice Nigeria.

Felner, E. (2009) 'Closing the "escape hatch": a toolkit to monitor the progressive realization of economic, social and cultural rights', *Journal of Human Rights Practice*, 1(3): 402–35.

Fernandez, K., and Koller, A. (2008) *Tabakpräventionsstrategie Steiermark: Jahresbericht 2008*, Graz: VIVID – Fachstelle für Suchtprävention: http://www.rauchfrei-dabei.at/de/service/downloads/tabakbericht (accessed June 2010).

Finnegan, A. C., Saltsman, A. P. and White, S. K. (2010) 'Negotiating politics and culture: the utility of human rights for activist organizing in the United States', *Journal of Human Rights Practice*, 2(3): 307–33.

Fisher, W. W., III and Rigamonti, C. P. (2005) 'The South Africa AIDS controversy: a case study in patent law and policy', in Harvard Law School, *The Law and Business of Patents*: http://cyber.law.harvard.edu/people/tfisher/South%20Africa.pdf (accessed Sept. 2011).

Flynn, M. M., Garkawe, S., and Holt, Y. (2011) *Human Rights: Treaties, Statutes and Cases*, Chatswood, NSW: LexisNexis Butterworths.

Ford, N., Calmy, A., and Hurst, S. (2010) 'When to start antiretroviral therapy in resource-limited settings: a human rights analysis', *BMC International Health and Human Rights*, 10(1).

Fox, A. M., and Meier, B. M. (2009) 'Health as freedom: addressing social determinants of global health inequities through the human right to development', *Bioethics*, 23(2): 112–22.

Fox, B. J. (2005) 'Framing tobacco control efforts within an ethical context', *Tobacco Control*, 14(suppl. 2): ii38–ii44.

FRA (2010a) *European Union Agency for Fundamental Rights Annual Report 2010, Conference Edition*, Vienna: FRA.

FRA (2010b) *Access to Justice in Europe: An Overview of Challenges and Opportunities*, Luxembourg: Publication Office of the EU.

FRA (2010c) *National Human Rights Institutions in the EU Member States: Strengthening the Fundamental Rights Architecture in the EU I*, Luxembourg: Publication Office of the EU.

Freeman, M. (1994) 'The philosophical foundations of human rights', *Human Rights Quarterly*, 16: 491–514.

Freire, P. (1972) *Pedagogy of the Oppressed*, London: Sheed & Ward.

Frisancho, A., and Goulden, J. (2008) 'Rights-based approaches to improve people's health in Peru', *The Lancet*, 372(9655): 2007–8.

Fry, C. L., Treloar, C., and Maher, L. (2005) 'Ethical challenges and responses in harm reduction research: promoting applied communitarian ethics', *Drug and Alcohol Review*, 24: 449–59.

Galvão, J. (2005) 'Brazil and access to HIV/AIDS drugs: a question of human rights and public health', *American Journal of Public Health*, 95(7): 1110–16.

García-Moreno, G., Jansen, H. A. F. M., Ellsberg, M., Heise, L., and Watts, C. (2005) *WHO Multi-Country Study on Women's Health and Domestic Violence Against Women*, Geneva: World Health Organization.

Gauri, V., Beyrer, C., and Vaillancourt, D. (2007) 'From human rights principles to public health practice: HIV/AIDS policy in Brazil', in C. Beyrer and H. F. Pizer (eds), *Public Health and Human Rights: Evidence Based Approaches*, Baltimore: Johns Hopkins University Press.

Gearty, C. (2006) *Can Human Rights Survive?* New York: Cambridge University Press.
Gesundheisförderung Schweiz (2009) *Ergebnismodell: Wirkungen systematisch planen und evaluieren*: www.gesundheitsfoerderung.ch/pages/Gesundheitsfoerderung_und_Praevention/Tipps_Tools/ergebnismodell.php (accessed Oct. 2009).
Ginbar, M. (2010) 'Human rights in ASEAN: setting sail or treading water?' *Human Rights Law Review*, 10(3): 504–18.
Glasier, A., and Gülmezoglu, A. M. (2006) 'Putting sexual and reproductive health on the agenda', *The Lancet*, 368: 1550–1.
Glasier, A., Gülmezoglu, A. M., Schmid, G. P., Moreno, C. G., and Van Look, P. F. A. (2006) 'Sexual and reproductive health: a matter of life and death', *The Lancet*, 368: 1595–1607.
Glasziou, P., and Longbottom, H. (1999) 'Evidence-based public health practice', *Australian and New Zealand Journal of Public Health*, 23(4): 436–40.
Gleeson, D. (2011) 'Trade agreement threatens health in Australia and Pacific', *Canberra Times*, editorial, 3 Aug.
GoI (2005) *Mid-Day Meal Scheme*: http://india.gov.in/sectors/education/mid_day_meal.php (accessed May 2010).
GoI (2008) *The Constitution of India*: http://lawmin.nic.in/coi/coiason29july08.pdf (accessed May 2010).
GOLD (2007) *GOLD – Generation Of Leaders Discovered: Annual Report 2007*, Rondebosch, Cape Town: GOLD.
GOLD (2008a) *Element 7: Monitoring and Evaluation*, Rondebosch, Cape Town: GOLD.
GOLD (2008b) *GOLD Exploratory Study: Identifying Direction of Potential Impact of GOLD PE Programme 2008*, Rondebosch, Cape Town: GOLD.
GOLD (n.d.) *GOLD Peer Education*, Rondebosch, Cape Town: GOLD: www.goldpe.org.za/about_gold.php (accessed May 2009).
Goldhaber, M. D. (2007) *A People's History of the European Court of Human Rights*, New Brunswick, NJ: Rutgers University Press.
Goldingay, S. (2007) 'Jail mums: the status of adult female prisoners among young female prisoners in Christchurch Women's Prison', *Social Policy Journal of New Zealand*, 31: 56–73.
Goldingay, S. (2009) 'Separation or mixing: issues for young women prisoners in Aotearoa New Zealand prisons', doctoral thesis, University of Canterbury, Social Work and Human Services, URI: http://hdl.handle.net/10092/3740.
Gostin, L., and Mann, J. (1994) 'Towards the development of a human rights impact assessment for the formulation and evaluation of health policies', *Health and Human Rights*, 1(1): 58–80.
Gostin, L. O., and Lazzarini, Z. (1997) *Human Rights and Public Health in the AIDS Pandemic*, New York: Oxford University Press.
Gostin, L. O., Friedman, E. A., Ooms, G., Gebauer, T., Gupta, N., Sridhar, D., Chenguang, W., Rttingen, J., and Sanders, D. (2011) 'The joint action and learning initiative: towards a global agreement on national and global responsibilities for health', *PLOS Medicine*, 8(5): e1001031.
Grech, O. (2009) 'Human rights and development', in C. Regan, B. Borg, and T. Meade (eds), *80:20 Development in an Unequal World*, Birmingham: Tide Global Learning.
Groene, O. (2011) 'Patient centredness and quality improvement efforts in hospitals: rationale, measurement, implementation', *International Journal for Quality in Health Care*, 23(5): 531–7.
Grover, A. (2010) *Report of the Special Rapporteur on the Right of Everyone to the Enjoyment of the Highest Attainable Standard of Physical and Mental Health*, Report to the 65th session of the UN General Assembly, A/65/255, New York: UN.

Grover, A. (2011) *Report of the Special Rapporteur on the Right of Everyone to the Enjoyment of the Highest Attainable Standard of Physical and Mental Health*, Report to the 66th session of the UN General Assembly, A/66/254, New York: UN.

Gruskin, S., and Daniels, N. (2008) 'Justice and human rights: priority setting and fair deliberative process', *American Journal of Public Health,* 98(9): 1573–7.

Gruskin, S., and Tarantola, D. (2001) 'HIV/AIDS, health, and human rights', in P. R. Lamptey and H. D. Gayle (eds), *HIV/AIDS Prevention and Care in Resource-Constrained Settings: A Handbook for the Design and Management of Programs*, Arlington, VA: Family Health International AIDS Institute.

Gruskin, S., and Tarantola, D. (2005) 'Health and human rights', in S. Gruskin, M. Grodin, S. Marks and G. Annas (eds), *Perspectives on Health and Human Rights*, New York: Routledge.

Gruskin, S., Grodin, M., Marks, S., and Annas, G., eds (2005) *Perspectives on Health and Human Rights*, New York: Routledge.

Gruskin, S., Ferguson, L., and Bogecho, D. O. (2007) 'Beyond the numbers: using rights-based perspectives to enhance antiretroviral treatment scale-up', *AIDS,* 21(suppl. 5): S13–19.

Gruskin, S., Mills, E. J., and Tarantola D. (2007) 'History, principles and practice of health and human rights', *The Lancet*, 370: 449–55.

Gruskin, S., Bogecho, D., and Ferguson, L. (2010) 'Rights-based approaches to health policies and programs: articulations, ambiguities, and assessment', *Journal of Public Health Policy*, 31(2): 129–45.

Gudavarthy, A. (2008) 'Human rights movements in India: state, civil society and beyond', *Contributions to Indian Sociology*, 42(1): 29–57.

Hargreaves, J., Hatcher, A., Busza, J., Strange, V., Phetla, G., Kim, J., Watts, C., Morison, L., Porter, J., Pronyk, P., and Bonell, C. (2011) 'What happens after a trial? Replicating a cross-sectoral intervention addressing the social determinants of health: the case of the Intervention with Microfinance for AIDS and Gender Equity (IMAGE) in South Africa', in E. Blas, J. Sommerfeld and A. S. Kurup (eds), *Social Determinants Approaches to Public Health: From Concept to Practice*, Geneva: WHO.

Harris, M., and Gartland, G. (2011) *Children of the Intervention: Aboriginal Children Living in the Northern Territory of Australia. A Submission to the UN Committee on the Rights of the Child*, Melbourne, Victoria: Concerned Australians.

Hawks, D., Scott, K., McBride, N., Jones, P., and Stockwell, T. (2002) *Prevention of Psychoactive Substance Use: A Selected Review of What Works in the Area of Prevention*, Geneva: World Health Organization.

Hazell, T. (2005a) *MindMatters: Evaluation of the Professional Development Program and School-level Implementation*, Newcastle, NSW: Hunter Institute of Mental Health.

Hazell, T. (2005b) 'Evaluating constructive solutions: implementation of MindMatters and evaluation of the professional development component', paper presented at 2005 AARE conference, Paramatta, NSW, Australia.

Health Canada (2003) *Canadian Guidelines for Sexual Health Education*, Ontario: Health Canada, Cat. N_ H39–300/2003E.

Hendriksen, E. S., Pettifor, A., Lee, S., Coates, T. J., and Rees, H. V. (2007) 'Predictors of condom use among young adults in South Africa: the reproductive health and HIV research unit national youth survey', *American Journal of Public Health*, 97: 1241–6.

Heywood, M. (2009) 'South Africa's treatment action campaign: combining law and social mobilization to realize the right to health', *Journal of Human Rights Practice*, 1(1): 14–36.

Hogerzeil, H. V., Samson, M., Casanovas, J. V., and Rahmani-Ocora, L. (2006) 'Is access to essential medicines as part of the fulfilment of the right to health enforceable through the courts?', *The Lancet*, 368: 305–11.

Holland, K. M. (2009) 'Rights protection in Japan: the political dimension', *Australian Journal of Political Science*, 44(1): 79–96.
Hopkins, D. P., Briss, P. A., Ricard, C. J., Husten, C. G., Carande-Kulis, V. G., Fielding, J. E., Alao, M. O., McKenna, J. W., Sharp, D. J., Harris, J. R., Woollery, T. A., and Harris, K. W. (2001) 'Reviews of evidence regarding interventions to reduce tobacco use and exposure to environmental tobacco smoke', *American Journal of Preventive Medicine*, 20(2): 16–66.
Hopkins, K. (2011) 'Amnesty International's methods of engaging youth in human rights education: curriculum in the United States and experiential learning in Burkina Faso', *Journal of Human Rights Practice*, 3(1): 71–92.
HRCl (2010) *Report of the Working Group on the Universal Periodic Review: Sweden, A/HRC/15/11*, New York: Human Rights Council.
HRW (2009) *Unbearable Pain: India's Obligation to Ensure Palliative Care*, New York: Human Rights Watch.
HRW (2011) *World Report: Events of 2010*, New York: Human Rights Watch.
Hunt, P. (2009) 'Missed opportunities: human rights and the Commission on Social Determinants of Health', *Global Health Promotion*, 1757–9(suppl. 1): 36–41.
Hunt, P., and MacNaughton, G. (2006) *Impact Assessments, Poverty and Human Rights: A Case Study Using the Right to the Highest Attainable Standard of Health*, Colchester: Human Rights Centre, University of Essex.
IACHR (2001) *Report No. 29/01 Case 12.249 Jorge Odir Miranda Cortez et al. El Salvador March 7, 2001*, Washington, DC: OAS.
IACHR (2009a) *Indigenous and Tribal Peoples' Rights over their Ancestral Lands and Natural Resources: Norms and Jurisprudence of the Inter-American Human Rights System*, Washington, DC: OAS.
IACHR (2009b) *Report No. 27/09 Case 12.249 Jorge Odir Miranda Cortez et al. El Salvador Merits Report, March 20, 2009*, Washington, DC: OAS.
IACHR (2010) *Access to Maternal Health Services from a Human Rights Perspective*, Washington, DC: OAS.
IACHR (2011) *Annual Report of the Inter-American Commission on Human Rights 2010*, Washington, DC: Inter-American Commission on Human Rights.
ICHRP, International Council on Human Rights Policy (2005) *Assessing the Effectiveness of National Human Rights Institutions*, Geneva: ICHRP/OHCHR.
Ife, J. (2008) *Human Rights and Social Work: Towards Rights Based Practice*, 2nd edn, Cambridge: Cambridge University Press.
Igras, S., Mutteshi, J., WoldeMariam, A., and Ali, S. (2004) 'Integrating rights-based approaches into community-based health projects: experiences from the prevention of female genital cutting project in East Africa', *Health and Human Rights*, 7(2): 251–71.
Iida, K. (2004) 'Human rights and sexual abuse: the impact of international human rights law on Japan', *Human Rights Quarterly*, 26(2): 428–53.
ILO (2011) *Freedom of Association and Development*, Geneva: ILO.
Ingleby, R., Prosser, L., and Waters, E. (2008) 'UNCROC and the prevention of childhood obesity: the right not to have food advertisements on television', *Journal of Law and Medicine*, 16 (1): 49–56.
Inter-American Court of Human Rights (2011) *Annual Report of the Inter-American Court of Human Rights 2010*, San Jose, Costa Rica: Organization of American States.
Ishay, M. R. (2008) *The History of Human Rights: From Ancient Times to the Globalization Era*, 2nd edn, Berkeley, CA: University of California Press.
ISHR (2011) *International Service for Human Rights Annual Report 2010*, Geneva: ISHR.

Itzin, C., Taket, A., and Barter-Godfrey, S. (2010a) *Domestic and Sexual Violence and Abuse: Findings from a Delphi Expert Consultation on Therapeutic and Treatment Interventions with Victims Survivors and Abusers, Children Adolescents and Adults*, Melbourne, Deakin University: www.dh.gov.uk/en/Publicationsandstatistics/Publications/PublicationsPolicyAndGuidance/DH_123971.

Itzin, C., Taket, A., and Barter-Godfrey, S., eds (2010b) *Domestic and Sexual Violence and Abuse: Tackling the Health and Mental Health Effects*, London: Routledge.

Jacobson, P. D., and Banerjee, A. (2005) 'Social movements and human rights rhetoric in tobacco control', *Tobacco Control*, 14(suppl. 2): ii45–ii49.

Jain, J., and Shah, M. (2005) 'Antyodaya Anna Yojana and Mid-day Meals in MP', *Economic and Political Weekly*, 40: 5076–88.

James, S., Reddy, P., Ruiter, R. A. C., McCauley, A., and Van Den Borne, B. (2006) 'The impact of an HIV and AIDS life skills program on secondary school students in Kwazulu-Natal, South Africa', *AIDS Education and Prevention*, 18: 281–94.

Jirasek, J. (2008) *Application of the Charter of Fundamental Rights of the EU in the United Kingdom and Poland according to the Lisbon Treaty*: www.law.muni.cz/sborniky/cofola2008/files/pdf/evropa/jirasek_jan.pdf (accessed May 2011).

Jones, L., Sumnall, H., Burrell, K., Mc-Veigh, J., and Bellis, M. A. (2006) *Universal Drug Prevention*, Liverpool: John Moores University, Centre for Public Health: www.drugpreventionevidence.info/documentbank/Universal.pdf (accessed March 2009).

Jonsson, U. (2003) *Human Rights Approach to Development Programming*, Nairobi: UNICEF.

Jürgens, R., and Cohen, J. (2007) *Human Rights and HIV/AIDS: Now More than Ever*, 2nd edn, New York: Open Society Institute.

Jürgens, R., Csete, J., Amon, J. J., Baral, S., and Beyrer, C. (2010) 'People who use drugs, HIV and human rights', *Lancet*, 376: 475–85.

Kagoiya, R., ed. (2009) *Freedom of Information and Women's Rights in Africa*, Nairobi: African Women's Development and Communication Network.

Kapoor, D. (2007) 'Gendered-caste discrimination, human rights education, and the enforcement of the prevention of atrocities act in India', *Alberta Journal of Educational Research*, 53(3): 273–86.

Katsumata, H. (2009) 'ASEAN and human rights: resisting western pressure or emulating the West?', *Pacific Review*, 22(5): 619–37.

Kaushik, S. K., Kaushik, S., and Kaushik, S. (2006) 'How higher education in rural India helps human rights and entrepreneurship', *Journal of Asian Economics*, 17(1): 29–34.

Kausikan, B. (1996) 'Asia's different standard', in H. J. Steiner and P. Alston (eds), *International Human Rights in Context*, Oxford: Clarendon Press.

Keane, H. (2003) 'Critiques of harm reduction, morality and the promise of human rights', *International Journal of Drug Policy*, 14: 227–32.

Keller, H., and Sweet, A. S., eds (2008) *The Reception of the ECHR in the Member States*, Oxford: Oxford University Press.

Kelsall, M. S. (2009) 'The new ASEAN intergovernmental commission on human rights: toothless tiger or tentative first step?', *Asia Pacific Issues*, 90: 1–8.

Kendall, T. (2009) 'Reproductive rights violations reported by Mexican women with HIV', *Health and Human Rights*, 11(2): 77–87.

Khoo, S-M. (2012) 'Re-interpreting the citizen consumer: alternative consumer activism and the rights to health and development', *Social Science and Medicine*, 74(1):14–9.

Kim, C. R., and Free, C. (2008) 'Recent evaluations for the peer-led approach in adolescent sexual health education: a systematic review', *International Family Planning Perspectives*, 34: 89–96.

Kinney, E. D. (2001) 'The international human right to health: what does this mean for our nation and world?', *Indiana Law Review*, 34(4): 1457–77.

Kinney, E. D. (2010) 'Realizing the international human right to health: the challenge of for-profit health care', *West Virginia Law Review*, 113: 49–66.

Koller, A. (2007) *Tabakpräventionsstrategie Steiermark: Jahresbericht 2007*, Graz: VIVID – Fachstelle für Suchtprävention: www.verwaltung.steiermark.at/cms/beitrag/11288205/21212 (accessed June 2010).

Krug, E. G., Dahlberg, L. L., Mercy, J. A., Zwi, A. B., and Lozano, R., eds (2002) *World Report on Violence and Health*, Geneva: World Health Organization.

Kufuor, K. O. (2010) *The African Human Rights System: Origin and Evolution*, New York: Palgrave Macmillan.

Kumar, C. R. (2006) 'National human rights institutions and economic, social and cultural rights: towards the institutionalization and developmentalization of human rights', *Human Rights Quarterly*, 28(3): 755–79.

Lage, A. (2011) 'Global pharmaceutical development and access: critical issues of ethics and equity', *MEDICC Review*, 13(3): 16–22.

Lam, W. K., Zhong, N. S., and Tan, W. C. (2003) 'Overview on SARS in Asia and the world', *Respirology*, 8(suppl.): S2–5.

Lazzarini, Z. (2003) 'Making access to pharmaceuticals a reality: legal options under TRIPS and the case of Brazil', *Yale Human Rights and Development Law Journal*, 6: 103–38.

Lecomte, J. and Mercier, C. (2008) 'The WHO atlas on global resources for persons with intellectual disabilities: a right to health perspective', *Salud Pública de México*, 50(suplemento 2): S160–S166.

Levinson, D., ed. (2003) *The Wilson Chronology of Human Rights*, New York: H. W. Wilson Co.

Lindsnaes, B., Lindholt, L., and Yigen, K., eds (2000) *National Human Rights Institutions: Articles and Working Papers*, Copenhagen: Danish Centre for Human Rights.

Lister-Sharp, D., Chapman, S., Stewart-Brown, S., and Sowden, A. (1999) 'Health promoting schools and health promotion in schools: two systematic reviews', *Health Technology Assessment*, 3(22): 1–207.

London, L. (2002) 'Human rights and public health: dichotomies or synergies in developing countries? Examining the case of HIV in South Africa', *Journal of Law, Medicine and Ethics*, 30: 677–91.

London, L. (2008) 'What is a human rights-based approach to health and does it matter?', *Health and Human Rights*, 10(1): 65–80.

Lovvorn, A. E., Quinn, S. C., and Jolly, D. H. (1997) 'HIV testing of pregnant women: a policy analysis', *Journal of Public Health Policy*, 18(4): 401–32.

Lülfs-Baden, F., and Spiller, A. (2009) 'Students' perceptions of school meals: a challenge for schools, school-meal providers, and policymakers', *Journal of Foodservice*, 20: 31–46.

Lülfs-Baden, F., Rojas-Méndez, J., and Spiller, A. (2008) 'Young consumers' evaluation of school meals', *Journal of International Food and Agribusiness Marketing*, 20: 25–47.

Lynch, P. (2009) 'Australia, human rights and foreign policy', *Alternative Law Journal*, 34(4): 218–26.

McBeth, A. (2004) 'Privatising human rights: what happens to the state's duties when services are privatised?', *Melbourne Journal of International Law*, 5: 133–54.

McClimans, L. M., Dunn, M., and Slowther, A.(2011) 'Health policy, patient-centred care and clinical ethics', *Journal of Evaluation in Clinical Practice*, 17(5): 913–19.

Macdonald, T. H. (2007) *The Global Human Right to Health: Dream or Possibility?*, Oxford: Radcliffe Publishing.

Macdonald, T. H. (2008) *Health, Human Rights and the United Nations: Inconsistent Aims and Inherent Contradictions?* Oxford: Radcliffe Publishing.

McHale, J. (2010) 'Fundamental rights and health care', in E. Mossialos, G. Permanad, R. Baeten and T. Hervey (eds), *Health Systems Governance in Europe: The Role of European Union Law and Policy*, Cambridge: Cambridge University Press.

MacNaughton, G., and Hunt, P. (2009) 'Health impact assessment: the contribution of the right to the highest attainable standard of health', *Public Health*, 123: 302–5.

MacNeil, C. (2011) *Making Local Government Work: An Activist's Guide*, South Africa: Section 27, Treatment Action Campaign and Read Hope Phillips: www.localgovernmentaction.org (accessed Sept. 2011).

Mandel, S. (2006) *Debt Relief as if People Mattered*, London: New Economics Foundation: www. neweconomics.org/publications/debt-relief-if-people-mattered (accessed Sept. 2011).

Manea, M. G. (2009) 'How and why interaction matters: ASEAN's regional identity and human rights', *Cooperation and Conflict*, 44(1): 27–49.

Mann, J. (1997) 'Medicine and public health, ethics and human rights', *Hastings Center Report*, 27(3): 6–13.

Mann, J., and Tarantola, D. (1998) 'Responding to HIV/AIDS: a historical perspective', *Health and Human Rights*, 2(4): 5–8.

Mann, J. M., Gostin, L., Gruskin, S., Brennan, T., Lazzarini, Z., and Fineberg, H. V. (1994) 'Health and human rights', *Health and Human Rights*, 1(1): 6–23.

Mann, J. M., Gostin, L., Gruskin, S., Brennan, T., Lazzarini, Z., and Fineberg, H. (1999) 'Health and human rights', in J. M. Mann, S. Gruskin, M. A. Grodin and G. J. Annas (eds) *Health and Human Rights: A Reader*, New York: Routledge.

Mann, S. (2004) '"Modernizing" the Arab Rights Charter', *Respect: The Human Rights Newsletter*, 20(201): 5.

Mapulanga-Hulston, J. K., and Harpur, P. D. (2009) 'Examining Australia's compliance to the International Covenant on economic, social and cultural rights: problems and potential', *Asia-Pacific Journal on Human Rights and the Law*, 10(1): 48–66.

Marks, S. P. (ed.) (2005) *Health and Human Rights: Basic International Documents*, Cambridge, MA: Harvard University Press.

Marmot, M. (2004) *Status Syndrome: How your Social Standing Directly Affects your Health*, London: Bloomsbury.

Martinez, A., and Phillips, K. P. (2008) 'Challenging ethno-cultural and sexual inequities: an intersectional feminist analysis of teachers, health partners and university students' views on adolescent sexual and reproductive health rights', *Canadian Journal of Human Sexuality*, 17(3): 141–60.

Mathiharan, K. (2003) 'The fundamental right to health care', *Indian Journal of Medical Ethics*, 11: 4.

Maticka-Tyndale, E., and Smylie, L. (2008) 'Sexual rights: striking a balance', *International Journal of Sexual Health*, 20(1–2): 7–24.

Mayhew, S., Douthwaite, M., and Hammer, M. (2006) 'Balancing protection and pragmatism: a framework for NGO accountability in rights-based approaches', *Health and Human Rights*, 9(2): 180–206.

Mayo, M., and Rooke, A. (2006) *Active Learning for Active Citizenship: An Evaluation Report*, London: Togetherwecan.

Mayo, M., and Rooke, A. (2008) 'Active learning for active citizenship: participatory approaches to evaluating a programme to promote citizen participation in England', *Community Development Journal*, 43(3): 371–381.

Meier, B. M. (2010) 'Global health governance and the contentious politics of human rights: mainstreaming the right to health for public health advancement', *Stanford Journal of International Law*, 46(1): 1–50.

Meijknecht, A., and De Vries, B. S. (2010) 'Is there a place for minorities' and indigenous peoples' rights within ASEAN? Asian values, ASEAN values and the protection of Southeast Asian minorities and indigenous peoples', *International Journal on Minority and Group Rights*, 17(1): 75–110.

Mertus, J. (2009) *The United Nations and Human Rights: A Guide for a New Era*, London and New York: Routledge.

Messer, E. (1993) 'Anthropology and human rights', *Annual Review Anthropology*, 22: 221–49.

Miller, S., and Hatamian, A. (2010) *Take Part Interim Report: Second Year Evaluation of the Take Part programme*, London: Community Development Foundation.

Ministry of Justice (n.d.) *Major Human Rights Problems*, Japanese Ministry of Justice: www.moj.go.jp/ENGLISH/HB/hb-03.html (accessed May 2010).

Mitchell, P. (2000) *Building Capacity for Life Promotion: Evaluation of the National Youth Suicide Prevention Strategy, Technical Report*, vol. 1, Melbourne: Australian Institute of Family Studies.

Mngadi, P. T., Faxelid, E., and Ransjo-Arvidson, A. B. (2008) 'Health providers' perceptions of adolescent sexual and reproductive health care in Swaziland', *International Council of Nurses*, 55: 148–55.

Moravcsik, A. (2000) 'The origins of human rights regimes', *International Organization*, 54(2): 217–52.

Morgaine, K. (2011) '"How would that help our work?": the intersection of domestic violence and human rights in the United States', *Violence Against Women*, 17(1): 6–27.

Morgan, R. E., and David, S. (2002) 'Human rights: a new language for aging advocacy', *Gerontologist*, 42(4): 436–42.

Moss, L. C. (2010) 'Opportunities for nongovernmental organization advocacy in the universal periodic review process at the UN Human Rights Council', *Journal of Human Rights Practice*, 2(1): 122–50.

Moyn, S. (2010) *The Last Utopia: Human Rights in History*, Cambridge, MA: Harvard University Press.

MSF (2010) *International Activity Report 2009*, Geneva: MSF.

Mujuzi, J. D. (2010) 'Michelot Yogogombaye v The Republic of Senegal: The African Court's First Decision', *Human Rights Law Review*, 10(2): 372–81.

Munro, J. (2009) 'Why states create international human rights mechanisms: the ASEAN intergovernmental commission on human rights and democratic lock-in theory', *Asia-Pacific Journal on Human Rights and the Law*, 10(1): 1–26.

Muntaner, C., Sridharan, S., Solar, O., and Benach, J. (2009) 'Commentary: against unjust global distribution of power and money. The report of the WHO commission on the social determinants of health: Global inequality and the future of public health policy', *Journal of Public Health Policy*, 30(2): 163–75.

Nagengast, C. (1997) 'Women, minorities, and indigenous peoples: universalism and cultural relativity', *Journal of Anthropological Research*, 53(3): 349–69.

Neshat, N. S. (2004) *Rights: Fourth Generation Human Rights? Human Rights in Information Society*, Teheran: Olive Leaf Publishing.

Neuwahl, N., and Rosas, A. (eds) (1995) *The European Union and Human Rights*, The Hague: Kluwer Law International.

NFI (2009) *Mid Day Meal Programme: A Historical Perspective*: www.nutritionfoundationofindia.res.in/Evaluation/Evaluation%20of%20%20Midady%20meal%20programme.pdf/Chapter%201%20_%20MDMP-A%20Historical%20Perspective_Evaluation%20of%20%20Midady%20meal%20programme_%20%20Pages%201-11.pdf (retrieved May 2010).

Ng, N.Y., and Ruger, J. P. (2011) 'Global health governance at a crossroads', *Global Health Governance*, 4(2): 1–37.

NHRC (2006) *The National Human Rights Commission, India*, New Delhi: NHRC.

NHRC (2009) *National Human Rights Commission, Annual Report 2007–2008*, New Delhi: NHRC.

Nixon, S., and Forman, L. (2008) 'Exploring synergies between human rights and public health ethics: a whole greater than the sum of its parts', *BMC International Health and Human Rights*, 8(special section): 1–9.

NTER Review Board (2008) *Northern Territory Emergency Response: Report of the NTER Review Board*, Canberra: Attorney General's Department.

Nunn, A., Da Fonesca, E., and Gruskin, S. (2009) 'Changing global essential medicines norms to improve access to AIDS treatment: lessons from Brazil', *Global Public Health*, 4: 131–49.

Nyamu-Musembi, C., and Cornwall, A. (2004) *What is the 'Rights-Based Approach' All About? Perspectives from International Development Agencies*, IDS Working Paper, 234, Brighton: Institute of Development Studies.

Nygren-Krug, H. (2003) *International Migration, Health and Human Rights*, Geneva: World Health Organization.

O'Brien, M. (2008) 'School meals: helping young bones', *British Journal of School Nursing*, 3: 278–80.

O'Flaherty, M., and Ulrich, G. (2010) 'The professionalization of human rights field work', *Journal of Human Rights Practice*, 2(1): 1–27.

OHCHR (n.d.) *The United Nations Human Rights System: An Introduction to the Core Human Rights Treaties and the Treaty Bodies. Fact Sheet 30*, Geneva: UN.

OHCHR (1993) *Principles Relating to the Status of National Institutions (The Paris Principles)*, UN General Assembly Resolution 48/134 of 20 Dec.

OHCHR (2000) *Business and Human Rights: A Progress Report*, Geneva: OHCHR.

OHCHR (2008) *Working with the United Nations Human Rights Programme: A Handbook for Civil Society*, Geneva: OHCHR.

OHCHR (2009a) *Survey on National Human Rights Institutions: Report on the Findings and Recommendations of a Questionnaire Addressed to NHRIs Worldwide*, Geneva: OHCHR.

OHCHR (2009b) *High Commissioner's Strategic Management Plan 2010–2011*, Geneva: OHCHR.

OHCHR (2011a) *OHCHR Report 2010*, Geneva: OHCHR.

OHCHR (2011b) *United Nations Special Procedures Facts and Figures 2010*, Geneva: OHCHR.

Oliver, S., and Peersman, G. (2002) *Using Research for Effective Health Promotion*, Philadelphia: Open University Press.

Ooms, G. (2011) *Global Health: What it Has Been So Far, What it Should Be, and What it Could Become*, Studies in Health Services Organisation and Policy, Working Paper, 2, Antwerp: Institute of Tropical Medicine.

Osei, A., Houser, R., Bulusu, S., and Hamer, D. (2008) 'Acceptability of micronutrient fortified school meals by schoolchildren in rural Himalayan villages of India', *Journal of Food Science*, 73: S354–8.

Osei, A., Rosenberg, I., Houser, R., Bulusu, S., Mathews, M., and Hamer, D. (2010) 'Community-level micronutrient fortification of school lunch meals improved vitamin A, folate, and iron status of schoolchildren in Himalayan villages of India', *Journal of Nutrition*, 140: 1146–54.

Pada, S., and Tambyah, P. A. (2011) 'Overview/reflections on the 2009 H1N1 pandemic', *Microbes and Infection*, 13(5): 470–8.

Paiva, V., Garcia, J., Rios, L. F., Santos, A. O., Terto, V., and Munoz-Laboy, M. (2010) 'Religious communities and HIV prevention: an intervention study using a human rights-based approach', *Global Public Health*, 5(3): 280–94.

Panter-Brick, C. (2002) 'Street children, human rights, and public health: a critique and future directions', *Annual Review of Anthropology*, 31: 147–71.

Peers, S., and Ward, A. (2004) *The EU Charter of Fundamental Rights: Politics, Law and Policy*, Oxford: Hart.

Pepin, G., Watson, J., Hagiliassis, N., and Larkin, H. (2010) 'Ethical and supported decision making', in K. Stagnitti, A. Schoo and D. Welch (eds), *Clinical and Fieldwork Placement in the Health Professions*, Melbourne: Oxford University Press.

Perkins, F. (2009) 'A rights-based approach to accessing health determinants', *Global Health Promotion*, 16(1): 61–4.

Pernice, I. (2008) *The Treaty of Lisbon and Fundamental Rights*, Walter Hallstein-Institut für Europäisches Verfassungsrecht Humboldt-Universität zu Berlin WHI-Paper 7/08: www.judicialstudies.unr.edu/JS_Summer09/JSP_Week_1/Pernice%20Fundamental%20Rights.pdf (accessed May 2011).

Pettifor, A. E., Kleinschmidt, I., Levin, J., Rees, H. V., MacPhail, C., Madikizela-Hlongwa, L., Vermaak, K., Napier, G., Stevens, W., and Padian, N. S. (2005) 'A community-based study to examine the effect of a youth HIV prevention intervention on young people aged 15–24 in South Africa: results of the baseline survey', *Tropical Medicine and International Health*, 10: 971–80.

PHM (2006) *The Assessment of the Right to Health and Health Care at the Country Level: A People's Health Movement Guide*, People's Health Movement: www.phmovement.org/files/RTH_assmt_tool.pdf (accessed Oct. 2011).

PIB (2010) *Mid-Day Meal Scheme*: http://pib.nic.in/archieve/flagship/bkg_mdm1.pdf (accessed May 2010).

Picard, M. (2005) *Principles into Practice: Learning from Innovative Rights-Based Programmes*, London: CARE International UK.

Pikkarainen, H., and Brodin, B. (2008a) *Discrimination of the Sami: The Rights of the Sami from a Discrimination Perspective*, Stockholm: Ombudsmannen mot etnisk diskriminering.

Pikkarainen, H., and Brodin, B. (2008b) *Discrimination of National Minorities in the Education System*, Stockholm: Ombudsmannen mot etnisk diskriminering.

Pillai, S., Seshu, M., and Shivdas, M. (2008) 'Embracing the rights of people in prostitution and sex workers, to address HIV and AIDS effectively', *Gender and Development*, 16(2): 313–26.

Pohjolainen, A. (2006) *The Evolution of National Human Rights Institutions: The Role of the United Nations*, Copenhagen: Danish Institute for Human Rights.

Prakasam, P. K., Vaidyanathan, K. E., Somayajulu, U. V., and Audinarayana, N., eds (2010) *Health, Equity and Human Rights: Perspectives and Issues*, New Delhi: Serials Publications/Indian Association for Social Sciences and Health.

Public Health Leadership Society (2002) *Principles of the Ethical Practice of Public Health*, New Orleans: Public Health Leadership Society.

PUCL (2010) *A Short History of PUCL*: www.pucl.org/history.htm (accessed May 2010).

Quashigah, E. K. (2000) 'The Ghana Commission on Human Rights and Administrative Justice', in B. Lindsnaes, L. Lindholt and K. Yigen (eds) (2000) *National Human Rights Institutions: Articles and Working Papers*, Copenhagen: Danish Centre for Human Rights.

Ramasubban, R. (2008) 'Political intersections between HIV/AIDS, sexuality and human rights: a history of resistance to the anti-sodomy law in India', *Global Public Health*, 3(suppl. 2): 22–38.

Rand, J., and Watson, G. (2008) *Rights-Based Approaches: Learning Project*, Boston, MA, and Atlanta, GA: Oxfam America and Care USA.

Rani, M., and Lule, E. (2004) 'Exploring the socioeconomic dimension of adolescent reproductive health: a multicountry analysis', *International Family Planning Perspectives*, 30: 110–17.

Rasanathan, K., Norenhag, J., and Valentine, N. (2010) 'Realizing human rights-based approaches for action on the social determinants of health', *Health and Human Rights*, 12(2): 49–59.

Rawls, J. (1971) *A Theory of Justice*, Oxford: Oxford University Press.

Rees, S. (2004) 'Human rights and the significance of psychosocial and cultural issues in domestic violence policy and intervention for refugee women', *Australian Journal of Human Rights*, 10(2): 19.

RHRU (2003) *HIV and Sexual Behaviour among Young South Africans: A National Survey of 15–24 Year Olds*, Johannesburg: University of the Witwatersrand.

Rid, A. (2009) 'Justice and procedure: how does "accountability for reasonableness" result in fair limit-setting decisions?', *Journal of Medical Ethics*, 35(1): 12–16.

Right to Food India (2010) *Mid-Day Meals: Supreme Court Order*: www. righttofoodindia. org/mdm/mdm_scorders.html (accessed May 2010).

Rishmawi, M. (2010) 'The Arab Charter on Human Rights and the League of Arab States: an update', *Human Rights Law Review*, 10(1): 169–78.

Rosoff, A. J. (1981) *Informed Consent: A Guide for Health Care Providers*, Rockville, MD: Aspen Systems Corporation.

Rostedt, A., and Vogel, J. (2009) *Report: Review of the Integration of a Human Rights-Based Approach and Gender Mainstreaming in Health Sector Planning and Processes in Yemen*, Cairo: WHO, Regional Office for Eastern Mediterranean.

Rowling, L. (1996) 'The adaptability of the health promoting schools concept: a case study from Australia', *Health Education Research*, 11(4): 519–26.

Rowling, L., Martin, G., and Walker, L., eds (2002) *Mental Health Promotion and Young People: Concepts and Practice*, Sydney: McGraw-Hill.

Royal College of Psychiatrists (2009) *Good Psychiatric Practice*, 3rd edn, *College Report CR154*, London: Royal College of Psychiatrists.

Ruger, J. P. (2010) *Health and Social Justice*, Oxford: Oxford University Press.

Samvad, V., Sanket, and Right to Food Campaign Madhya Pradesh Support Group (2009) *Moribund ICDS: A Study on the ICDS and Child Survival Issues in Madhya Pradesh*, Bhopal: Authors.

Sanchez Fuentes, M. L., Paine, J., and Elliott-Buettner, B. (2008) 'The decriminalisation of abortion in Mexico City: how did abortion rights become a political priority?', *Gender and Development*, 16(2): 345–60.

SAPA TFAHR (2010) *Hiding behind its Limits: A Performance Report of the First Year of the ASEAN Intergovernmental Commission on Human Rights 2009–2010*, Bangkok: Forum-Asia, Asian Forum for Human Rights and Development.

SARC (2011) *Review of the Charter of Human Rights and Responsibilities Act 2006*, Melbourne: Parliament of Victoria.
Sarelin, A. L. (2007) 'Human rights-based approaches to development cooperation, HIV/AIDS, and food security', *Human Rights Quarterly*, 29(2): 460–88.
Sarin, E., Samson, L., Sweat, M., and Beyrer, C. (2011) 'Human rights abuses and suicidal ideation among male injecting drug users in Delhi, India', *International Journal of Drug Policy*, 22(2): 161–6.
Saxena, N.C. (2002) *Food Assistance Programmes and their Role in Alleviating Poverty and Hunger in India*: www.sccommissioners.org/pdfs/Articles/foodassistanceprogrammessaxena.pdf (accessed May 2010).
SEARO (2011) *The Right to Health in the Constitutions of Member States of the World Health Organization South-East Asia Region*, New Delhi: WHO, Regional Office for South-East Asia.
Sen, A. (1999) *Development as Freedom*, New York: Random House.
Sen, A. (2009) *The Idea of Justice*, London: Penguin.
Shade, L. R. (2004) 'Situating communication rights historically', in M. Moll and L. R. Shade (eds), *Seeking Convergence in Policy and Practice: Communications In the Public Interest*, vol. 2, Ottawa: Canadian Centre for Policy Alternatives.
Shaikh, H. (2009) 'OIC to set up independent human rights commission', *The Saudi*, 14 May: www.saudigazette.com.sa (accessed May 2011).
Sharma, A. (2006) *Are Human Rights Western?: A Contribution to the Dialogue of Civilizations*, New Delhi: Oxford University Press.
Sharma, S. (2003) 'Human rights of mental patients in India: a global perspective', *Current Opinion in Psychiatry*, 16(5): 547–51.
Sheehan, M., Cahill, H., Rowling, L., Marshall, B., Wynn, J., and Holdsworth, R. (2002) 'Establishing a role for schools in mental health promotion: the MindMatters project', in L. Rowling, G. Martin and L. Walker (eds), *Mental Health Promotion and Young People: Concepts and Practice*, Sydney: McGraw-Hill.
Shestack, J. J. (1998) 'The philosophic foundations of human rights', *Human Rights Quarterly*, 20: 201–34.
Shin, H. S. (2001) 'Review of school-based drug-prevention program evaluation in the 1990s', *American Journal of Health Education*, 32: 139–47.
Short, J. L. (1998) 'Evaluation of a substance abuse prevention and mental health promotion program for children of divorce', *Journal of Divorce and Remarriage*, 28: 139–55.
SHRC (2009) *Human Rights in a Health Care Setting: Making it Work*, Glasgow: Scottish Human Rights Commission.
Silva, M.-L. (2003) *The Human Rights Based Approach to Development Cooperation towards a Common Understanding among UN Agencies*, Geneva: Office of the High Commissioner for Human Rights.
Simbayi, L. C., Kalichmann, S. C., Jooste, S., Cherry, C., Mfecane, S., and Cain, D. (2005) 'Risk factors for HIV-AIDS among youth in Cape Town, South Africa', *AIDS and Behaviour*, 9: 53–61.
Simonelli, F., and Fernandes Guerreiro, A. I. (2010) *Final Report on the Implementation Process of the Self-Evaluation Model and Tool on the Respect of Children's Rights in Hospital*, Florence: International Network of Health Promoting Hospitals and Health Services.
Simmons, B. (2002) *Why Commit? Explaining State Acceptance of International Human Rights Obligations*, Cambridge, MA: Weatherhead Center for International Affairs, Harvard University.
Singh, A. (2008) *Do School Meals Work? Treatment Evaluation of the Midday Meal Scheme in India*. Oxford: Young Lives Student Paper.

Singh, A. (2010) 'Commentary: rights-based approaches to health policies and programmes. Why are they important to use', *Journal of Public Health Policy*, 31(2): 146–9.

Singh, J. A., Govender, M., and Mills, E. J. (2007) 'Do human rights matter to health?', *The Lancet*, 370: 521–7.

Sripati, V. (2000) 'India's National Human Rights Commission: strengths and weaknesses', in B. Lindsnaes, L. Lindholt and K. Yigen (eds), *National Human Rights Institutions: Articles and Working Papers*, Copenhagen: Danish Centre for Human Rights.

Statistics Austria (2010a) *Total Population (Annual Average)*: www.statistik.at/web_en/statistics/population/population_stock_and_population_change/total_population_annual_average/index.html (accessed June 2010).

Statistics Austria (2010b) *International Migrations*: www.statistik.at/web_en/statistics/population/migration/internal_migration/index.html (accessed June 2010).

Stewart-Brown, S. (2006) *What is the Evidence on School Health Promotion in Improving Health or Preventing Disease and, Specifically, What is the Effectiveness of the Health Promoting Schools Approach?* Copenhagen: WHO Regional Office for Europe: www.euro.who.int/document/e88185.pdf.

Stiglitz, J. (2006) *Making Globalisation Work*, Harmondsworth: Penguin.

Stuttaford, M., Hundt, G. L., and Vostanis, P. (2009) 'Sites for health rights: the experiences of homeless families in England', *Journal of Human Rights Practice*, 1(2): 257–76.

Sub-Commission on the Promotion and Protection of Human Rights (2001) *The Impact of the Agreement on Trade-Related Aspects of Intellectual Property Rights on Human Rights*, UN Doc. E/CN.4/Sub.2/2001/13, Geneva: UN.

Surjadjaja, C., and Mayhew, S. H. (2011) 'Can policy analysis theories predict and inform policy change? Reflections on the battle for legal abortion in Indonesia', *Health Policy and Planning*, 26(5): 373–84.

Swaminathan, M. (2008) *Programmes to Protect the Hungry: Lessons from India*, Working Papers, 70, New York: United Nations, Department of Economics and Social Affairs.

Taket, A. (2012) 'Health and social justice', in P. Liamputtong, R. Fanany and G. Verrinder (eds), *Health, Illness and Well-Being: Perspectives and Social Determinants*, Melbourne: Oxford University Press.

Taket, A. R., Crisp, B. R., Nevill, A., Lamaro, G., Graham, M., and Barter-Godfrey, S. (2009) *Theorising Social Exclusion*, London: Routledge.

The Advocates for Human Rights (2011) *The Advocates for Human Rights 2010 Annual Report*, Minneapolis: The Advocates for Human Rights.

't Hoen, E. (2005) 'TRIPS, pharmaceuticals, patents and access to essential medicines: a long way from Seattle to Doha', in S. Gruskin, M. Grodin, S. Marks and G. Annas (eds) *Perspectives on Health and Human Rights*, New York: Routledge.

Tilley, J. J. (2000) 'Cultural Relativism', *Human Rights Quarterly*, 22(2): 501–47.

Tiwana, M., Aurora, S., and Punj, A. (2006) *Human Rights Commissions: A Citizen's Handbook*, New Delhi: Commonwealth Human Rights Initiative.

Tolley, M. C. (2009) 'Parliamentary scrutiny of rights in the United Kingdom: assessing the work of the Joint Committee on Human Rights', *Australian Journal of Political Science*, 44(1): 41–55.

Tones, K., and Green, J. (2004) *Health Promotion: Planning and Strategies*, London: Sage.

Trubek, D. M., and Trubek, L. G. (2005) 'Hard and soft law in the construction of social Europe: the role of the open method of co-ordination', *European Law Journal*, 11(3): 343–64.

Tsutsui, K., and Shin, H. J. (2008) 'Global norms, local activism, and social movement outcomes: global human rights and resident Koreans in Japan', *Social Problems*, 55(3): 391–418.

Turiano, L., and Smith, L. (2008) 'The catalytic synergy of health and human rights: the People's Health Movement and the Right to Health and Health Care Campaign', *Health and Human Rights*, 10(1): 137–47.

Uhl, A., Bachmayer, S., and Kobrna, U. (2009) 'Chaos um die Raucherzahlen in Österreich (Chaos concerning smoking prevalence figures in Austria)', *WMW Wiener Medizinische Wochenschrift*, 159(1): 4–13.

UN (1945) *Charter of the United Nations and Statute of the International Court of Justice*, New York: UN.

UN Centre for Human Rights (1994–1997) *Human Rights: A Compilation of International Instruments*, New York: UN.

UN General Assembly (1948) *Universal Declaration of Human Rights, UN Doc. A/810*, New York: UN.

UN General Assembly (1965) *International Convention on the Elimination of All Forms of Racial Discrimination, UN Doc. A/RES/2106 (XX)*, New York: UN.

UN General Assembly (1966a) *International Covenant on Economic, Social and Cultural Rights, UN Doc. A/RES/2200(XXI)*, New York: UN.

UN General Assembly (1966b) *International Covenant on Civil and Political Rights, UN Doc. A/RES/2200(XXI)*, New York: UN.

UN General Assembly (1979) *Convention on the Elimination of All Forms of Discrimination Against Women, UN Doc. A/RES/34/180*, New York: UN.

UN General Assembly (1989) *Convention on the Rights of the Child, UN Doc. A/RES/44/25*, New York: UN.

UN General Assembly (1993) *Report of the World Conference on Human Rights: Report of the Secretary-General*, A/CONF.157/24 (Part I), New York: UN.

UN General Assembly (2010) *Promotion and Protection of Human Rights, Including Ways and Means to Protect the Human Rights of Migrants, Report of the Secretary-General*, A/65/156, New York: UN.

UN Secretary-General (2011) *Uniting For Universal Access: Towards Zero New HIV Infections, Zero Discrimination and Zero AIDS Related Deaths, Report of the Secretary-General*, A/65/797, New York: UN.

UN Women (2011) *Progress of the World's Women 2011–2012: In Pursuit of Justice*, New York: UN Women.

UNEP (2011) *Environmental Assessment of Ogoniland*, Nairobi: UNEP.

UNFPA (1994) *Programme of Action: adopted at the International Conference on Population and Development*, Cairo, 5–13 Sept.: www.unfpa.org/icpd/icpd-programme.cfm#ch7e (accessed Aug. 2009).

UNFPA and Harvard School of Public Health (2010) *A Human Rights-Based Approach to Programming: Practical Information and Training Materials*, New York: UNFPA.

Vencatesan J. (2008) 'The next good meal', *Current Science*, 94: 12.

Venkatapuram, S., Bell, R., and Marmot, M. (2010) 'The right to sutures: social epidemiology, human rights, and social justice', *Health and Human Rights*, 12(2): 3–16.

VEOHRC (2010a) *Annual Report 2009/10*, Melbourne: VEOHRC.

VEOHRC (2010b) *Talking Rights: Consulting with Victoria's Indigenous Community about the Right to Self-Determination and the Charter*, Melbourne: VEOHRC.

VEOHRC (2010c) *Talking Rights: Consulting with Victorians about the Rights of People with Disabilities and the Charter*, Melbourne: VEOHRC.

VEOHRC (2010d) *Talking Rights: Consulting with Victorians about Economic, Social and Cultural Rights and the Charter*, Melbourne: VEOHRC.

VEOHRC (2010e) *Advancing Women's Rights: Exploring the Relationship between the Charter of Human Rights and Responsibilities and the Convention on the Elimination of All Forms of Discrimination Against Women*, Melbourne: VEOHRC.

VEOHRC (2011a) *Talking Rights: 2010 Report on the Operation of the Charter of Human Rights and Responsibilities*, Melbourne: VEOHRC.

VEOHRC (2011b) *Talking Rights: Compilation Report. Resource Materials to Accompany the 2010 Report on the Operation of the Charter of Human Rights and Responsibilities*, Melbourne: VEOHRC.

VEOHRC (2011c) *Parliamentary Review of the Victorian Charter of Human Rights: 14 Sep 2011*, Melbourne: VEOHRC: www.humanrightscommission.vic.gov.au/index.php?option=com_k2&view=item&id=1493:parliamentary-review-of-the-victorian-charter-of-human-rights-14-sep-2011&Itemid=3 (accessed Oct. 2011).

Victorian Health Promotion Foundation (2004) *The Health Cost of Violence: Measuring the Burden of Disease Caused by Intimate Partner Violence*, Melbourne: Victorian Health Promotion Foundation.

VIVID (2010) *Newsletter*, Sept.: www.rauchfrei-dabei.at/de/newsletter/newsletter_september (accessed Feb. 2011).

Wakefield, M. K. (1997) 'Protecting health care consumers: a bill of rights and responsibilities', *Nursing Economics*, 15(2): 110–11.

Wallerstein, N. (2006) *What is the Evidence on Effectiveness of Empowerment to Improve Health?* Copenhagen: WHO Regional Office for Europe (Health Evidence Network report: www.euro.who.int/__data/assets/pdf_file/0010/74656/E88086.pdf. Accessed October 2011).

Wang, Z., and Hoy, W. (2005) 'Albuminuria and incident coronary heart disease in Australian Aboriginal people', *Clinical Science*, 99(3): 247–51.

Ward, T., and Moreton, G. (2008) 'Moral repair with offenders: ethical issues arising from victimization experiences', *Sexual Abuse: Journal of Research and Treatment*, 20(3): 305–22.

Wearing, M. (2011) 'Strengthening youth citizenship and social inclusion practice: the Australian case. Towards rights based and inclusive practice in services for marginalized young people', *Children and Youth Services Review*, 33(4): 534–40.

White, S., Park, Y. S., Israel, T., and Cordero, E. D. (2009) 'Longitudinal evaluation of peer health education on a college campus: impact on health behaviours', *Journal of American College Health*, 57: 497–505.

Whitehead, M. (1990) *The Concepts and Principles of Equity in Health, Discussion Paper*, Copenhagen: World Health Organization, Regional Office for Europe.

WHO (1986) *Ottawa Charter for Health Promotion*, 1st International Conference on Health Promotion, Ottawa: WHO, WHO/HPR/HEP/95.1.

WHO (1997) *Violence Against Women: A Health Priority Issue, FRH/WHD/97.8*, Geneva: WHO.

WHO (2001) *International Classification of Functioning, Disability and Health*, Geneva: WHO.

WHO (2002a) *25 Questions and Answers on Health and Human Rights*, Geneva: WHO: www.who.int/hhr/activities/publications/en.

WHO (2002b) *The Right to Health*, Geneva: WHO.

WHO (2003a) *HIV/AIDS: Stand up for Human Rights*, Geneva: WHO.

WHO (2003b) *WHO Framework Convention on Tobacco Control*, Geneva: WHO.

WHO (2007a) *The Gambia: Effective and Humane Mental Health Treatment and Care for All*, Geneva: WHO.

WHO (2007b) *WHO Guidelines on Human Rights and Involuntary Detention for Extensively Drug-Resistant Tuberculosis Control*, Geneva: WHO: www.who.int/tb/features_archive/involuntary_treatment/en/index.html (accessed May 2011).

WHO (2008a) *The Right to Health: Fact Sheet 31*, Geneva: WHO.

WHO (2008b) *Human Rights, Health and Poverty Reduction Strategies*, Geneva: WHO/OHCHR.

WHO (2010) *HIV/AIDS: Stand up for Human Rights*, updated edn, Geneva: WHO.

WHO (2011) *Human Rights and Gender Equality in Health Sector Strategies: How to Assess Policy Coherence*, Geneva: WHO.

WHO/UNAIDS (2006) *Progress on Global Access to HIV Antiretroviral Therapy: A Report on '3 by 5' and Beyond*, Geneva: WHO.

Wild, R., and Anderson, P. (2007) *Ampe Akelyernemane Meke Mekarle: Little Children are Sacred. Report of the Northern Territory Board of Inquiry into the Protection of Aboriginal Children from Sexual Abuse*, Darwin: Northern Territory Government.

Wilkinson, R., and Marmot, M. (2003) *Social Determinants of Health: The Solid Facts*, Copenhagen: European Regional Office, WHO.

Wolfe, D., and Malinowska-Sempruch, K. (2007) 'Seeing double: mapping contradictions in HIV prevention and illicit drug policy worldwide', in C. Beyrer and H. F. Pizer (eds), *Public Health and Human Rights: Evidence Based Approaches*, Baltimore, MD: Johns Hopkins University Press.

Woodward, V. (2004) *Active Learning for Active Citizenship*, London: Home Office.

World Health Assembly (2000) *HIV/AIDS: Confronting the Epidemic, Resolution WHA53:14*, Geneva: WHO.

Worm, I. (2010) *Human Rights and Gender Equality and Health: Overview of Impact Assessment Tools*, Health and Human Rights Working Paper Series, 7, Geneva: WHO: www.who.int/hhr/information/papers/en/index.html.

Yen, Y.-M. (2011) 'The formation of the ASEAN Intergovernmental Commission on Human Rights: a protracted journey', *Journal of Human Rights*, 10(3): 393–413.

Zarsky, L., ed. (2002) *Human Rights and the Environment: Conflicts and Norms in a Globalizing World*, London: Earthscan.

Index

acceptability 17, 18, 80, 109
access 17, 18, 48, 52, 63, 92, 111, 122, 123, 131, 142–4, 147; campaign about 28, 31, 32, 84–5, 165; to essential medicines 1, 28, 31, 45, 71, 75, 81, 82–5, 157, 160, 163–4, 167–8; to health care 16, 31, 45, 50, 52, 59, 60, 65, 75–7, 85, 106, 113, 137, 143, 163, 168; to human rights system 29, 42, 47, 50, 69, 71; to information 17, 18, 27, 31, 136, 138; to services 31, 45, 47, 48, 52, 75, 89, 98, 115, 140, 148, 157, 163–4, 166, 168
accessibility 17, 18, 19, 80, 96, 109, 153
accession 11
accountability 5, 79, 80, 104, 111, 148, 153; Accountability for Reasonableness 152–5; accountability of duty-bearers 77; accountability of governments 5, 59, 63, 161–2; accountability of NGOs 87, 88, 92, 119, 145; accountability of private sector 34; accountability of service providers 92, 124, 128, 138
Active Learning for Active Citizenship (ALAC) 95, 96–9, 101, 157–8, 159, 162
advocacy 1, 4–6, 16, 44, 62, 77, 82, 87, 100, 101, 115, 147, 148, 150, 154, 162; by NGOs 24, 27–9, 30–1, 31, 49, 65, 77, 89, 165; policy advocacy 80, 81–5, 162; by special rapporteurs 25
Afghanistan 70
Africa 4, 30, 35–40, 57, 69, 73, 86, 114, 115, 168, 169, 170–1; Central Africa 23; East Africa 23, 91; Southern Africa 23; West Africa 23
African Charter on Human and Peoples' Rights (Banjul Charter) 35, 36, 37, 39
African Commission on Human and Peoples' Rights (ACHPR) 36, 37, 38, 39, 40, 170

African Court on Human and Peoples' Rights 36, 38, 39, 171
African Union 35, 36, 37, 38, 39, 171
AICHR, see ASEAN Intergovernmental Commission on Human Rights
AIDS see HIV/AIDS
Alma Ata declaration 17, 19, 31, 165
America, Americas 4, 35, 36, 40–8, 55, 57, 69, 73, 91, 171; Central America 23, 72; Latin America 44, 72, 81, 162; South America 23
American Convention on Human Rights 36, 40–1, 43
Amnesty International 27–9, 101, 165–6, 170
Annan, Kofi 164
antiretroviral therapy or antiretrovirals (ARV) 45, 46, 75, 81, 82, 84–5, 103, 105, 115, 157
Arab Charter on Human Rights 36, 53
Arab Region 23, 36, 53–4, 171
Argentina 31, 41, 69, 72
ASEAN, see Association of South East Asian Nations
ASEAN Intergovernmental Commission on Human Rights (AICHR) 36, 48–9, 167
Asia 4, 35, 36; Central Asia 23; South-East Asia 20, 23, 73; South-West Asia 23
Asia-Pacific 4, 48–9, 57, 69, 70, 91, 171
Association of Southeast Asian Nations (ASEAN) 32–3, 36, 48–9, 171
asylum seekers 6, 27, 63, 163, 164; see also refugees
Australia 4, 5, 25–7, 28, 33, 57, 60–4, 69, 70, 71, 76, 77, 78–9, 93, 103, 112, 139–45, 151, 154, 159, 162, 172
Australian Human Rights Commission (AHRC) 60–1, 69, 172
Austria 5, 52, 76, 103, 112, 130–8, 159

availability 17, 18, 65, 66, 80, 83, 84, 124, 132, 157

Ban, Ki-moon 30
Bangladesh 31, 49, 73, 87, 91, 165
Barbados 41
Belarus 77
Belgium 28, 31
Belize 11
Bhutan 73
Bolivia 41, 87
Brazil 31, 41, 76, 81–6, 92, 157
Brunei Darussalam 48
Burkina Faso 38, 101
Burundi 25, 87

Cairo Declaration on Human Rights in Islam 36, 53, 54
Cairo Institute for Human Rights Studies (CIHRS) 54, 171
Cambodia 25, 48, 49, 87, 91
Canada 15, 103, 158
capacity building 70, 89, 90, 96, 114, 156, 157, 159
cardiovascular disease (CVD) 151
CARE International 80, 86–91, 92, 101, 158, 159, 160, 162, 169, 172
carers 92, 97
Caricom 30
Center for Reproductive Rights 28, 31, 162, 168
Charter of Fundamental Rights of the European Union 36, 51, 171
Chile 23, 41, 168
citizen 11, 31, 41, 51, 53, 58, 85, 86, 90, 95, 97, 127, 168
citizenship 68, 95–9, 136
civil society 31, 49, 57, 73, 85, 87, 91, 92, 158, 162, 168, 169
climate change 33, 168
coercion/coercive treatment 75, 107, 109, 115, 118, 127
Colombia 30, 41, 81
Commission on Human Rights 8, 19, 23
Commission on Human Rights and Administrative Justice (CHRAJ) 59–60, 70, 172
Commission on the Social Determinants of Health (CSDH) 2, 147–50
Committee Against Torture (CAT) 12, 22
Committee on Economic, Social and Cultural Rights (CESCR) 16, 22, 146, 152

Committee on Enforced Disappearance (CED) 22
Committee on the Elimination of Discrimination against Women (CEDAW) 22, 76
Committee on the Elimination of Racial Discrimination (CERD) 22, 63
Committee on the Protection of the Rights of All Migrant Workers and Members of their Families (CMW) 22–3
Committee on the Rights of the Child (CRC) 22
Committee on the Rights of Persons with Disabilities 22
communication 21, 22, 25, 26, 38, 39, 40, 41; see also complaint
Comoros 11
complaint 22, 23, 27, 36, 41, 45, 55, 57, 58, 60, 61, 62, 64, 93, 111, 119, 124, 138, 168; see also communication
Convention Against Torture and other Cruel, Inhuman or Degrading Treatment or Punishment (CAT) 12, 22, 70, 167
Convention on the Elimination of All Forms of Discrimination Against Women (CEDAW) 12, 16, 22, 48, 76, 137, 167, 168
Convention on the Rights of the Child (CRC) 12, 13, 16, 22, 33, 48, 49, 137, 144, 162, 167
Convention on the Rights of Persons with Disabilities (CRPD) 10, 12, 16, 22, 33, 70
core obligations 17, 146, 160, 163
Costa Rica 36, 41, 43
Council of Europe 36, 49, 52
Covenant on the Rights of the Child in Islam 36, 54
Croatia 69
Cuba 11, 15, 157
Czech Republic 51

debt relief 161
Democratic People's Republic of Korea 25, 73
determinants of health 17, 18, 20, 92, 159, 160; see also social determinants of health
development 13, 18, 32, 37, 49, 79, 86, 87, 91, 157, 161, 165, 166, 167; health development 19, 75, 77, 158
disabled people 6, 37, 67, 95, 98, 163; see also people/persons with disabilities
disadvantaged groups 1, 2, 3, 6, 18, 66, 78, 89, 91, 103, 112, 119, 122, 123, 124,

129, 150–5, 158, 159, 164, 166; *see also* marginalised groups, vulnerable groups
domestic violence 45, 60, 75, 76, 93, 98, 142
Dominica 41
Dominican Republic 41
drug use 75, 77, 92, 139, 158; *see also* substance abuse
duty-bearers 77, 87, 88, 90, 92, 159, 161, 166

Ecuador 41, 69, 72
education 2, 8, 9, 10, 11, 20, 21, 37, 41, 48, 52, 54, 58, 59, 61, 75, 78, 80, 81, 92, 100, 121–9, 139–45, 147, 151, 158; *see also* health education, human rights education, peer education, right to education
El Salvador 41, 46, 69
employment 8, 21, 52, 58, 60, 61, 75, 78, 86, 97, 112, 123, 125, 127, 129
empowerment 1, 46, 79, 80, 87, 89, 92, 95–101, 106, 114, 117, 120, 125, 156, 159
England 81, 91, 168
environment 10, 11, 13, 16, 17, 33, 37, 39, 41, 51, 88, 95, 102, 136, 146, 165
Equality and Human Rights Commission (EHRC) 81, 82, 92–3
equity 2–3, 18, 44, 87, 90–1, 96, 103, 106, 112, 125–6, 128, 142, 158, 160; *see also* health equity
essential medicines 1, 18, 28, 31, 65, 71, 81, 82–5, 157, 164, 167
Ethical Guidelines for Biomedical Research 44
ethics 2, 3, 17, 18, 32, 44, 94–5, 106, 125, 148, 149–50; medical ethics 17, 18, 44; professional ethics 32, 94, 95; public health ethics 94
Ethiopia 38, 91
ethnic groups/minorities 3, 9, 12, 18, 38, 47, 52, 58, 59, 93, 109, 136, 158
Europe 4, 23, 35, 36, 49–52, 57, 69, 83, 84, 92, 93, 133, 150, 169, 171
European Commission 52
European Convention on Human Rights (ECHR) 36, 49, 50, 51, 52, 72, 81, 167
European Court of Human Rights 36, 49, 50, 51, 52, 94
European Union (EU) 32, 36, 49, 51, 52, 73, 84, 171
European Union Agency for Fundamental Rights (FRA) 52, 73

Fiji 91

first-generation rights 9, 11
food 2, 8, 9, 17, 20, 21, 39, 41, 48, 75, 86, 87, 121–9, 147, 162
food quality 48, 124, 125, 128
for-profit enterprises 81
fourth-generation rights 9, 13
France 28, 31
freedom of expression 8, 9, 10, 11, 13, 14, 21, 50, 53, 58, 60, 62, 151
freedom of movement 8, 11, 13, 14, 15, 21, 41, 62, 63, 76, 108, 109, 118
freedom of speech 118, 145
Freire, Paulo 97

Gabon 31
Gambia 35, 36, 40
Ghali, Boutros Boutros 7, 32
Ghana 4, 31, 57, 59–60, 70, 86, 172
gender 11, 18, 26, 27, 53, 58, 59, 61, 66, 80, 86, 88, 90, 93, 97, 100, 102, 108, 112, 122, 125, 128, 132, 158, 159, 168
gender-based violence 45, 47, 115
General Comment 21, 152, 163; General Comment 3 on 'The nature of States parties' obligations' 17, 152; General Comment 14 on 'The right to health' (GC 14) 16, 17, 19, 20, 109, 136, 146, 160, 163
Germany 28
governance 4, 54, 60, 69, 79, 88, 89, 98, 165, 167, 169
Grenada 41
Guatemala 41, 87

Haiti 25, 41
harm reduction 6, 75, 77, 162
health education 116, 136, 158
health equity 2–3, 4–5, 21, 75–101, 129, 163, 167
health promotion 19, 106, 118, 129, 131, 138, 144, 149, 150; advocacy 16; foundations of 1, 156; human rights approach to 86, 158; mental health promotion 5, 139, 140, 142, 144, 145; planning 130
Health Rights of Women Assessment Instrument (HeRWAI) 102, 157, 160
HIV/AIDS 1, 5, 6, 15, 18, 19, 20, 45, 46, 80, 81, 82–6, 91, 92, 96, 100, 103, 111, 113–20, 147, 157, 158, 160, 164, 165, 168, 169
HIV prevention 82, 92, 103, 105, 111, 113–20, 168
Honduras 41, 87

housing 8, 17, 52, 63, 78, 81, 97; *see also* shelter
Human Rights Committee (HRC) 22, 25–7, 51
Human Rights Council (HRCl) 23, 24, 25, 67, 70, 84
Human Rights and Equal Opportunities Commission (HREOC) 60, 69, 70
human rights, key features of 9–10; human rights analysis 1, 2, 5, 6, 20, 90, 102, 103, 104, 106, 111, 113–45, 149, 152, 158; human rights defenders 29, 58, 68, 168; human rights education 34, 73, 80, 95, 96, 100–1, 157, 168; human rights impact assessment 80, 102, 103, 148; *see also* rights
Human Rights Watch (HRW) 28, 29, 30–1, 65

India 4, 5, 31, 33, 49, 57, 64–6, 69, 70, 72, 73, 75, 82, 87, 88, 91, 92, 100, 103, 112, 121–9, 159, 165, 169, 172
indigenous people 12, 13, 18, 25, 32, 33, 45, 47, 48, 49, 59, 67, 75; indigenous Australians 33, 63–4, 78–9, 144, 151–4; Maori 33; Pacific Islander 33; Sami 59
Indonesia 48, 49, 70, 73, 91
infectious disease 15; *see also* HIV/AIDS, SARS, tuberculosis
intellectual property 82, 83, 84, 85
intellectual property rights (IPR) 82, 83
Inter-American Commission on Human Rights (IACHR) 36, 40–8, 76, 171
Inter-American Court of Human Rights 36, 40–3, 171
Inter-Governmental Organisation or International Governmental organisation (IGO) 23, 38, 53, 54
International Classification of Functioning, Disability and Health (ICFDH) 95
International Conference on Population and Development (ICPD) 113, 163
International Convention on the Elimination of All Forms of Racial Discrimination (ICERD) 12, 16, 22, 137, 167
International Convention on the Protection of the Rights of All Migrant Workers and Members of Their Families (ICRMW) 12, 16, 22
International Coordinating Committee of National Human Rights Institutions (ICC) 57, 68–70
International Council on Human Rights Policy (ICHRP) 73

International Covenant on Civil and Political Rights (ICCPR) 9–14, 22, 25, 61, 118, 127, 151, 154, 155, 167
International Covenant on Economic, Social and Cultural Rights (ICESCR) 9–14, 16, 17, 19, 20, 22, 61, 83, 127, 136, 146, 154, 167, 168
International Labour Office (ILO) 169
International Service for Human Rights (ISHR) 28, 29
Ireland 28, 69

Jamaica 41
Japan 4, 49, 57, 66–8, 70, 166, 172
Jordan 69, 70

Kenya 69, 91

Lao PDR 48, 91
lesbian, gay, transsexual, bisexual and intersexual (LGTBI) 26, 27, 30–1, 46, 47, 58, 59; *see also* sexual minorities, sexuality
Luxembourg 69

Mahler, Halfdan 19
Malaysia 48, 49, 70, 165
Maldives 73
mandate-holder 24–5
Mann, Jonathan 19, 20, 103
marginalised groups 1, 18, 32, 86, 87, 88, 90, 91, 99, 129, 159, 160, 166; *see also* disadvantaged groups, vulnerable groups
Médecins Sans Frontières (MSF) 28, 31, 84, 170
mental health 5, 16, 25, 37, 40, 44, 93, 97, 103, 112, 139–45, 146; mental health services 40, 44, 63, 93, 95
Mexico 41, 69, 162
Middle East 4, 23, 35, 36, 53–4, 171
migrant workers 12, 22, 49, 97–8
migrants 6, 97, 106, 112, 136
MindMatters, 5, 103, 112, 139–45
minorities 12, 18, 32, 33, 48–9, 53, 59; *see also* ethnic minorities, sexual minorities
Mongolia 49, 70
monitoring and reporting systems, global 21–7
Morocco (Maroc) 54, 69
Myanmar 25, 48, 49, 73

National Human Rights Commission (NHRC) 64–6, 69, 70, 165, 172

National Human Rights Institution (NHRI) 4, 24, 34, 35, 52, 56–8, 66–7, 68–70, 71, 73–4, 81, 93, 166, 168, 172; NHRI network 57, 68–70
negative rights 11
Nepal 49, 70, 73, 91
Netherlands 31
New Zealand 33, 69, 70
Nicaragua 41
Nigeria 37, 39
non-governmental organisation (NGO): involvement in the global system 10, 21, 24, 27–32, 34, 76, 77, 84–5, 170; involvement in regional systems 35, 38, 48, 49, 53, 67, 68, 76; and RBAs 86–91, 92, 95, 165, 168
Northern Ireland 93, 95
Northern Territory Emergency Response (NTER) 64, 78–9
Norway 28, 31
Niger Delta Region 37, 39
nutrition 17, 20, 51, 66, 75, 88–9, 121–9

Office of the United Nations High Commissioner for Human Rights (OHCHR) 12, 14, 17, 21–5, 34, 35, 47, 57, 69–70, 73, 79, 100, 168, 170
Ogoni people 39
Optional Protocol to the Convention Against Torture (OPCAT) 12, 70
Organisation of Islamic Cooperation (formerly Organisation of the Islamic Conference) (OIC) 4, 30, 36, 54, 171
Organization of African Unity (OAU) 35, 37, 38, 84
Organization of American States (OAS) 36, 40, 41, 43, 171
Ottawa charter 2
over-inclusion 103, 107, 108, 126, 137, 142, 143

Pacific 23, 167; *see also* Asia-Pacific
Pakistan 49, 92
Palestinian territories 25, 70
Pan American Health Organization (PAHO) 43, 44–5, 55
palliative care 65
Panama 23, 41, 44
Paraguay 41
Paris Principles 56–7, 69, 70, 71, 73
patient-centred care 94, 157
People's Health Movement (PHM) 28, 31–2, 102, 160, 165

People's Union for Civil Liberties (PUCL) 121
peer education 101, 103, 111, 113–20
people with disabilities 63; *see also* disabled people, persons with disabilities
Permanent Arab Commission on Human Rights (PACHR) 36, 53
person-centred approaches 94
persons with disabilities 10, 12, 18, 22, 33, 51, 70, 160; *see also* disabled people, people with disabilities
Peru 41, 87, 91
pharmaceutical companies 81, 82, 83, 85
Philippines 32, 48, 49, 70, 91
Pillay, Navi 26, 27, 34
Poland 51
pollution *see* environment
pornography 25, 67
positive rights 11, 73
poverty 6, 46, 47, 86–7, 88, 91, 122, 147, 151, 160, 161, 169
power 3, 64, 65, 66, 68, 91, 101; power relations 6, 79, 90, 91, 101, 103, 108, 109, 157, 159
professional standards 94
prisoners 28, 33, 50, 67, 81, 85, 92
private sector 18, 34, 60, 62, 66, 81, 82, 87, 118, 126
prostitution 25, 67, 92
public health 2, 8, 16, 19, 39, 73, 80, 82, 146; and domestic violence 76; as grounds for restriction or limitation of rights 10, 13, 14, 15, 109–10; and intellectual property rights 82–5; practice 1, 4–5, 19–20, 94, 150, 151; practitioners 1, 84, 102, 111, 149; programmes, human rights analysis of 102, 106, 108, 113–20, 121–9, 130–8, 139–45; value of human rights for 6, 16, 38, 62, 66, 83, 156–69

quality of life 46, 65, 94, 133; quality of services 17, 18, 80, 93, 109, 114, 144

rape 45
ratification 11, 20, 21, 36, 39, 41, 48, 49, 59, 63, 64, 71, 109
refugees 6, 12, 63, 76, 91, 151–4, 163, 164; *see also* asylum seekers
reproductive health 1, 6, 17, 20, 31, 45, 86, 94, 113–20, 151, 157, 158, 163–4
resource allocation 6, 123, 150, 152, 154, 155, 166, 168

right to education 8, 9, 10, 13, 20, 21, 37, 41, 61, 75, 80, 127, 137, 144
right to health 4, 80, 109, 118, 121, 127, 135, 136, 137, 138, 142, 146, 148, 149, 151, 155; campaigns for 85, 91, 165, 169; challenges to achievement of 167; definitions in ICESCR and GC14 16–20; for-profit sector and 81; in Arab charter on Human Rights 53; in Banjul Charter 37; in Protocol of San Salvador 41; lack of in ECHR 50; manuals/guides to 94, 96, 100, 158, 168; progress towards achievement of 20, 38, 44, 50, 65–6, 71–3, 77, 156,160, 164; recognition of at national level 20, 57, 65–6, 71–3; tools for assessing progress towards 102, 160, 163
right to health care: in European Charter of Fundamental Rights 52, 85, 102, 160, 165
right to information 13, 18, 75, 80, 89, 93, 108, 109, 128, 137, 151
right to life 8, 9, 10, 41, 46, 50, 51, 62, 64, 65, 121, 127
right to privacy 8, 11, 25, 26, 41, 62, 75, 80, 103, 106, 109
rights: absolute rights 10; civil and political rights 9–13, 22, 41, 61, 64, 81, 118, 127; economic, social and cultural rights 9–13, 22, 28, 29, 39, 41, 46, 47, 63, 64, 81, 83, 90, 127, 136, 146, 152, 156, 159, 168; first-generation rights 9, 11, 13; fourth-generation rights 9, 13, 33, 87; limitation of rights 10, 13–15, 53, 106, 109, 144; negative rights 11; positive rights 11; relative rights 10; reproductive rights 28, 31, 68, 113, 162, 164, 165, 168; restriction of rights 10, 13–15, 20, 64, 75, 102, 104, 106–10, 112, 118, 127, 137, 143, 144, 147, 164, 168; second-generation rights 9, 11, 13; third-generation rights 9, 13; *see also* human rights
rights-based approach (RBA) 1, 2, 4–6, 19, 77–80, 81, 82, 85, 86–93, 94–5, 95–101, 102, 118, 147, 150, 156–69
rights-holders 77, 87, 88, 90, 159
rights of children 33, 54, 58, 60, 63, 67, 93, 135, 137, 138, 140; *see also* CRC
rights of indigenous people 12, 13, 25, 33, 45, 47, 49, 59, 63, 64, 67, 75, 78–9, 154
rights of migrant workers 12, 22, 49, 97–8
rights of persons with disabilities 10, 12, 22, 33, 51, 63, 70, 160
rights of women 12, 22, 25, 33, 45, 47, 48, 49, 54, 60, 63, 67, 68, 75, 76, 88, 102–3, 113, 135, 137, 138, 157, 160, 163, 165, 169
Robinson, Mary 16
Roosevelt, Eleanor 8, 95
Rwanda 30, 87

sanitation 17, 18, 21
Sao Tome and Principe 11
Scotland 93, 95
Scottish Human Rights Commission (SHRC) 93, 95
Scrutiny of Acts and Regulations Committee (SARC) 63
second-generation rights 9, 11, 13
severe acute respiratory syndrome (SARS) 15, 107–8
sex work *see* prostitution
sex workers 92, 106, 108
sexual health 6, 17, 20, 31, 94, 113–20, 157, 158, 164
sexual minorities 52; *see also* lesbian, gay, transsexual, bisexual and intersexual (LGTBI)
sexuality 25–7, 92, 93, 100, 101, 108, 117, 158
sexually transmissible infection (STI) 85, 108, 113, 115, 116, 164
shelter 2, 8, 9, 21, 39, 75, 87, 147; *see also* housing
Sierra Leone 87
Singapore 48, 49
signature 11, 13
Siracusa principles 13, 15, 80, 109, 110, 118, 127, 144
slavery 8, 9 10, 20, 68, 75
social determinants of health 1, 2–3, 4, 5, 20–1, 37, 75, 86, 112, 141, 147–50, 155, 156, 159, 160, 167, 169
social exclusion 46, 47, 88
social fragility 81
social justice 2–4, 5, 6, 11, 35, 77, 86, 95, 96, 148, 149, 150, 152, 165, 169
social mobilisation 30, 85, 87, 100, 158, 169
social movement 28, 31, 32, 33, 66, 93, 100, 102, 160, 165
social work 94, 95
Solidarity for Asian People's Advocacy Task Force on ASEAN and Human Rights (SAPA TAFHR) 48, 49
Somalia 25, 87

South Africa 5, 11, 30–1, 69, 72, 73, 83–4, 85, 94, 103, 111, 113–20, 158, 159, 169
South Korea (Republic of Korea) 49, 70
Special Procedures 23, 24–5,
Special Rapporteur 25, 30, 77, 147, 162, 164
Sri Lanka 49, 73
stakeholder 5, 24, 27, 73, 79, 87, 88, 92, 93, 99, 101, 108, 111, 118, 119, 131, 133, 153, 159; stakeholder analysis 101
strengths-based approaches 94, 156
substance use/abuse 115; *see also* drug use
Sudan 25
Suriname 30, 41
Sweden 4, 28, 57, 58–9, 70, 71, 171

Taiwan 49
Tanzania 36, 38
Thailand 48, 49, 70, 73, 77, 87
third-generation rights 9, 13
Timor Leste 49, 70, 73
tobacco prevention 5, 103, 112, 130–8
Togo 69
Toonen, Nick 25–7
torture 8, 9, 10, 11, 12, 17, 20, 22, 28, 30, 32, 38, 50, 62, 70, 75
Trade-Related Aspects of Intellectual Property Rights (TRIPS) 83–5
trafficking 25
treaty bodies 21, 22, 23, 24, 69, 152, 162, 166
tuberculosis 107–8, 164

Uganda 30, 86
UNAIDS the Joint United Nations Programme on HIV/AIDS 82, 84, 100
under-inclusion 103, 107, 108, 126, 137, 143
United Kingdom (UK) 28, 31, 51, 71, 72, 81, 86, 92–6, 106, 157, 172; *see also* England, Northern Ireland, Scotland, Wales
United Nations Children's Fund (UNICEF) 47, 86, 157, 158
United Nations Development Programme (UNDP) 84
United Nations Environment Programme (UNEP) 39

United States (USA) 11, 28, 30, 32, 41, 71, 84, 91, 93, 101
Universal Declaration of Human Rights (UDHR) 1, 4, 7–10, 13, 14, 16, 28, 33, 40, 53, 61, 66, 70, 82, 94, 95, 109, 127, 136, 141, 143, 146
Universal Periodic Review (UPR) 23, 24, 59, 63, 67, 70, 79, 162
universality 9, 32
Uruguay 41

Venezuela 41, 44, 81
Victorian Charter of Rights and Responsibilities 61, 62
Victorian Equal Opportunity and Human Rights Commission (VEOHRC) 61, 62, 63, 172
Vietnam 48
violence against women *see* gender-based violence
vulnerable groups 18, 57, 66, 80, 91, 92, 94, 97, 108, 114, 117, 119, 129, 136, 152, 154, 158, 159, 166; *see also* disadvantaged groups, marginalised groups

Wales 81, 92
water 17, 18, 21, 39, 48, 86, 87, 122, 128
WHO Eastern Mediterranean Regional Office (EMRO) 101
WHO Regional Office for Africa (AFRO) 40
WHO Regional Office for Europe (EURO) 133, 169
WHO Regional Office for South-East Asia (SEARO) 20, 73
Women's Global Network for Reproductive Rights (WGNRR) 28, 31–2, 165
World Health Assembly (WHA) 19, 84, 160
World Health Organization (WHO) 6, 16, 17, 18, 19, 20, 40, 44, 55, 73, 77, 79, 80, 82, 84, 91, 95, 96, 100, 102, 133, 146, 147, 149, 156–60, 163, 164, 169
World Trade Organization (WTO) 82–5, 167

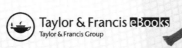